THE EXPERII BEING AN AUTISTIC FOSTER CARE GIVER WORKING WITH UK SOCIAL SERVICES

Megan Tanner

THE EXPERIENCES OF BEING AN AUTISTIC FOSTER CARE GIVER WORKING WITH UK SOCIAL SERVICES

"I Thought There was Something Wrong with Her..."

The Disability Studies Collection

Collection Editors
**Dr Jennifer Smith-Merry
& Dr Damian Mellifont**

First published in 2024 by Lived Places Publishing

All rights reserved. No part of this publication may be reproduced, stored in a retrieval system, or transmitted in any form or by any means, electronic, mechanical, photocopying, recording or otherwise, without prior permission in writing from the publisher.

The authors and editors have made every effort to ensure the accuracy of information contained in this publication, but assume no responsibility for any errors, inaccuracies, inconsistencies, or omissions. Likewise, every effort has been made to contact copyright holders. If any copyright material has been reproduced unwittingly and without permission the Publisher will gladly receive information enabling them to rectify any error or omission in subsequent editions.

Copyright © 2024 Lived Places Publishing

British Library Cataloguing in Publication Data
A CIP record for this book is available from the British Library

ISBN: 9781915734716 (pbk)
ISBN: 9781915734723 (ePDF)
ISBN: 9781915734730 (ePUB)

The right of Megan Tanner to be identified as the Author of this work has been asserted by her in accordance with the Copyright, Design and Patents Act 1988.

Cover design by Fiachra McCarthy
Book design by Rachel Trolove of Twin Trail Design
Typeset by Newgen Publishing UK

Lived Places Publishing
Long Island
New York 11789

www.livedplacespublishing.com

Abstract

How can social workers and neurodiverse foster carers collaborate to provide the best support for a child or teen in need? Building strong relationships between social workers and neurodiverse foster carers can be challenging. Drawing from her own lived experience as a neurodivergent foster carer, Megan Tanner explains how a successful partnership can create the best possible outcome. Working to remove pre-conceptions and judgement surrounding neurodiverse foster carers, this book is ideal reading for students and practitioners of social work and related courses, disability studies, autism and autistic studies, DEIB studies, psychology, and social work policy makers.

Keywords

Lived experience; DEIB; social work; policy; mental health; anxiety; neurodiversity; relationships; communication; trust

Contents

Introduction		ix
Learning objectives		xix
Chapter 1	The benefits of autistic foster carers	1
Chapter 2	Perceptual differences	15
Chapter 3	Executive functioning differences	31
Chapter 4	Social differences	43
Chapter 5	Truth differences	59
Chapter 6	Rule differences	85
Chapter 7	Autistic overwhelm	99
Conclusion		111
Recommended assignments and discussion questions		131
References		132
Recommended further reading		139
Glossary		140
Index		145

Trigger warning

This book contains explicit references to, and descriptions of, situations which may cause distress. This includes references to and descriptions of:

- Ableism, discrimination, and micro-aggressions

Please be aware that references to potentially distressing topics occur frequently and throughout the book.

Introduction

When I told people I was a foster carer the usual response was, "Wow. I bet that is so rewarding", or "How wonderful. What a valuable job you do".

I would give a positive reply because I really did love fostering, and my children and my teenagers. It was rewarding. There was another truth, though. I was also broken by an organisation that could not or would not accept my difference, my neurodivergence, and refused to make any reasonable adjustments. I love being autistic. No matter what I faced I would not change being autistic for anything.

My diagnosis

I started my journey with fostering in 2011 and in August 2019 was diagnosed as being autistic. I would love to say that, when my local authority and fostering agency found out, they sat me down and asked what reasonable adjustments I felt would be helpful, or that they challenged their assumptions and decisions about me now that I had an official diagnosis. But no. I was told I needed to redo my medical immediately!

For what? How could the results change now that I had an official diagnosis of autism? I was the same person as I had been in 2011. I had not changed. I refused and asked them to check the legality of their request! I was not asked to take the medical again, thankfully.

It has been said, "If you have met 1 autistic person you have met 1 autistic person", and this is very true. Autism is not linear as some believe, it is a spectrum, and we all have different attributes within it. So, in writing this book I can only use my experiences. I am not able to assume those of others (that is part of my autism). The lived experience examples and stories are mine and I hope they will go towards helping the system understand ways in which they can be more inclusive for neurodivergent foster carers.

It has only been in the past few years that autism has become more widely understood and diagnosed. I was born in 1978 and, even though I displayed traits during my childhood, autism was never considered as a reason for my behaviour. Autism is also less frequently diagnosed in females.

> Many more boys than girls are diagnosed on the autism spectrum: more than four boys for every autistic girl, according to the latest numbers from the Centers for Disease Control. Researchers point to genetic differences. But clinicians and researchers have also come to realize that many "higher functioning" autistic girls are simply missed. They've been termed the "lost girls" or "hiding in plain sight" because they're overlooked or diagnosed late. They don't fit the stereotypes or their symptoms are misinterpreted as something else. And they may be better at hiding the signs, at least when they're young.
>
> (Arky, 2023)

This could mean that there are a lot of adults who are autistic and undiagnosed within the foster carer community, especially females. If we can understand "difference", we can make the workplace environment better for all people, diagnosed or undiagnosed.

It is important to note that, when I started my fostering journey, I did explain that there was a GP's suggestion that I was autistic, and I was waiting to have an assessment. For the first few years I did not have a diagnosis. However, as you will see, my behaviours were pretty obvious. A quote I often repeat in various situations is, "If it quacks like a duck, it is a duck". I was clearly a duck. So, in 2011, I presented as an autistic person, and, in 2019, I was proved to be an autistic person. Social services were fully aware of the waiting lists and how costly it was to go privately for an assessment. Clearly, the understanding should have been that getting a full diagnosis was going to take years and that should have been an important fact in my file. However, as we can see throughout this book, prior to and following the diagnosis in August 2019, nothing in their attitude showed any understanding of autism and how it would present. Whether I was "suspected" or "fully diagnosed" it did not matter. Nothing was put in place to alleviate any difficulties I faced with the organisation.

I believe social services, as it was called when I started fostering, is now known in the UK as social care. I struggle with this concept of "care", so until I hear and see that it is a "care" system and not a "service" system I will continue to call it social services. The experiences I describe in this book are not those of a system geared to "care".

Celebration of exceptional social workers

I do not want this to appear to be all negative. I do want to celebrate the positive people and times too. Sadly, these positive contributions only help to highlight the difficult and negative issues. Many things could have been different. They did not need to be the way they were. The memories of these outstanding social workers prove this. In an email from my first supervising social worker, just before we went into a meeting I was anxious about, I was told that they had not been informed whether XX would be attending or not. However, it continued, if that is the case, "pls, pls, pls hold fire", and to let them do the talking. They explained that they may seem a bit slow in putting things forward but it was usually better to allow others in the forum to speak and then present your case! They promised they were still supporting my application to become a long-term foster carer and they were also confident that the application would be approved. They clearly understood that I would find the process tedious but they reiterated that it was their job to take any pressure off. They even told me to turn to them during periods of distress … and, if it would help, give them a sharp kick under the table to release any frustration! They thanked me and explained that they truly valued and appreciated my time, energy, and commitment to this and they were so glad that I was sticking with it despite the initial challenges! They continued, "You're fab to work with … and it's not me who's a superior worker but you!!! I'm so sorry that it's taken time for your efforts to be openly recognized. Look forward to seeing you later.)"

They knew I struggled with a certain manager and that I became very anxious with this manager's "communication techniques". So, they gave me the tools to help. They encouraged and supported me; used humour, reminded me that I was not alone in this meeting, they were there, and they had my back and best interests at heart. They would do their job. They enabled me to be relaxed without heading into fight or flight mode when walking into the meeting.

I only had two supervising social workers during my years as a foster carer. This is a blessing as both of mine were amazing. The chapters in this book are meant to highlight issues, but I do want to say I have had a few good people behind me during my fostering journey, and, although supervising social workers do not have that much power when problematic issues arise within the system, they are invaluable. Being able to use them as supporters, to talk to, to vent on, to know there is one person at least who knows you, understands you, and is on your side means the world. So, to E and A, if you ever read this book, thank you!

When it comes to child social workers I cannot remember how many I had over the years. It must be in the tens. The turnover was fast. Many were agency workers who only dipped in for a week or so to the detriment of the children and young people they were there to help. Good as they may have been, they could not make effective change in their short-term intervention.

I remember one child social worker from years ago in particular. By the time she came along I had enough years of fostering under my belt to be wary and protective, both of myself and the children and young people in my care. However, she shattered my defences within a short time by being utterly child focused.

She would pop over on her way home long after her working hours had finished. She understood that the "normal" methods we were told to do in parenting sessions were not working with our child. We had a meeting and she allowed me to find and try ideas that could work. For this I am so thankful! She related to me as someone who had worth. I never felt "less than", difficult, or simply a work appointment. She celebrated small wins. She knew that, on some days, due to the extreme behaviours our child was displaying, I would be drained, even feeling like I could not do it any longer, and she would tell me to go make a coffee while she sat with our child and gave me a break. When she found out I had left fostering I received this:

> Such a shame, maybe you will foster again when the time is right. You are an amazing carer, and I will never forget what you stepped up to do for "X". Big hugs.
>
> (Child social worker, personal communication)

This was years after our child had moved on in the system. Neither of us worked for that local authority any more. It would have been completely acceptable for her to have forgotten me. I know she would have had her fair share of foster carers in the interim. This message meant, and still means, so much to me.

So, yes, I have had child social workers who were legends, who reduced the stress levels of living with and parenting highly traumatised children and young people who played out their trauma in their behaviours. They relit my candle flame when I was exhausted. If ever you read this book, then thank you, S, for being incredible!

The sad problem is that social workers like E, A, and S were few and far between. These are three truly exceptional social workers in 11 years out of goodness knows how many. Many were too tired, overworked, or afraid to stand against the norm for the children they were there for. Despite their best efforts they could not change the system, even if they tried. And that is what is needed – but that is another book!

Survival mode

> I think if you keep people in survival mode, and you keep them in fear, and you keep them at War, and you keep them angry, and you keep them in pain, and you keep them confused you can control their attention by controlling their emotions.
>
> (Dispenza in Bartlett, 2023)

When I heard this quote it reminded me of being a foster carer. I was in survival, I was in fear, I was angry, I was hurt, and I was confused. My attention was constantly on where the next unexpected, disappointing issue was coming from with the adults. But I should have been relaxed, happy, worthy in my role in social services so I could look after my children and young people with no other pressures. My question is why does the system want or need their foster carers to be in this position? What is going on? If something does not make sense, then something is going on that is not right. Would we even dare to scratch the surface of that suggestion? Would it even matter if we did? After all, Ofsted pronouncements of failings can go on for years, even decades, with no real positive change happening. And that is an easily verifiable fact.

For balance, it can be a postcode lottery with regards to how foster carers are treated. I am sure there are local authorities who actually do equality and inclusion well.

Parenting

Parenting for anyone, whether neurotypical or neurodivergent, is difficult, exhausting, and stressful. For foster carers, add into the mix the need to face extreme trauma, neglect, abuse, adverse childhood experiences, child on parent violence, challenging, violent, or dangerous behaviour, child sexual exploitation, verbal aggression, high risk activity, defiance, self-harm, dysregulation, absconding, police visits, drugs and alcohol misuse, school issues, rape, sleep difficulties, foetal alcohol syndrome – the list goes on. Parenting goes to the next level of "difficult". Fostering is emotionally draining for anyone.

We need a system, true social care, which appreciates that we, as foster carers, live with these children continuously. We do not clock in at 9 a.m. and out at 5 p.m., with weekends and annual holidays off. We deserve a social care system which desires to support us so we can parent the children and young people in our care with no added stress.

If this book is able to make a change, then let that be the change. Support us, accept us, believe in us, and celebrate us. Be the organisation that refuses to add unnecessary stress onto humans who are actually in the arena. Become social care and not social services.

So, what does this book look like?

Each chapter of this book goes through an aspect of my autism, how it presents in me, and the difficulties I had as a foster carer with many of the adults within the system. I have used actual, lived experience examples from my years as a foster carer, then, at the end of each chapter, I have suggested a few reasonable adjustments that can easily be made. The term "reasonable adjustments" and any other specific terms I have used are explained in the Glossary.

The Equalities Act 2010 means neurodivergent people are "protected" within the work environment and it is illegal for any employer not to make reasonable adjustments to help us at work. The National Autistic Society states: "Employers are legally obliged to support you and make reasonable adjustments" (2023).

> Employers can be required by law to make reasonable adjustments to the workplace. Failure to do so may be discrimination.
> Adjustments should respond to the particular needs of the worker. Examples of adjustments include changes to work premises, changes to work schedules, modifying equipment or providing training.
> (Australian Human Rights Commission, 2023)

These reasonable adjustments are in no way comprehensive but hopefully they will spark ideas.

This book itself shows how this is so often neglected and, when it is flagged as a problem, nothing is done about it. This needs to change! Not only for neurodivergent carers but for all if we are to see retention of foster carers and less burnout in those working within social services.

xviii   Experiences of Being an Autistic Foster Care Giver

Social services needs to comply and make reasonable adjustments. As I have said it is not difficult to create a safer environment for carers. It just needs to be something which is actually wanted and it can be done.

I hope this book helps you understand and include "difference" and gives you some ideas on how to be inclusive.

I want to say to you the words of Michelle Obama: "Don't ever underestimate the importance you can have because history has shown us that courage can be contagious and hope can take on a life of its own" (Gajanan, 2017).

So read this book and go out and be the change we need.

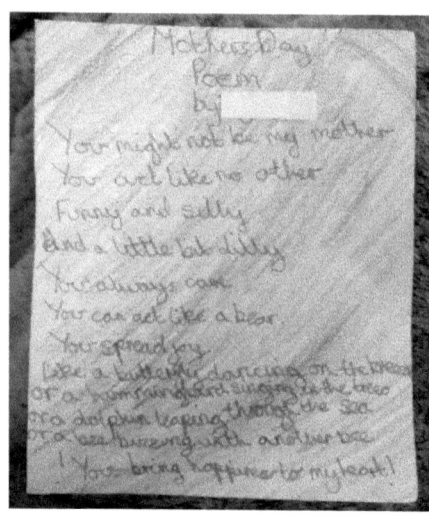

Figure 1

Learning objectives

1. To understand difference.
2. To question our personal judgements and prejudices.
3. To see the added value neurodivergence brings.
4. To be unafraid of different communication styles.
5. To be able to implement reasonable adjustments.

1
The benefits of having autistic foster carers

Why might autistic people make good foster carers?

Let's be positive and start with the benefits of being an autistic foster carer. These are numerous. The chapters in this book are going to look at all of the issues which actually arose from my being autistic, so, for balance, we need to understand what autistic foster carers can bring to fostering.

In a study on "The Strengths and Abilities of Autistic People in the Workplace": "The main strengths identified from this data revealed cognitive advantages such as superior creativity, focus, and memory; increased efficiency and personal qualities such as honesty and dedication; and the ability to offer a unique autism-specific perspective" (Cope and Remington, 2022).

In parenting my autism has huge benefits. Here are a few from the top of my head. Any stories I add throughout the book are from my own lived experiences, or those of my tribe who are now in their adult years, out of the care system and who have given permission for me to use them. Most examples will be about me as this is about my autism and the effects on my fostering journey, but this section will need a few about my tribe as they were an integral part of the whole experience.

My autism allowed me, as a foster carer, to create routines which were immovable. This may sound counterproductive, but, in fact, as the children and teenagers I fostered were highly traumatised, they needed the stability of routine as this helped them feel secure. Routines did not change; I did not flipflop; they were safe.

My autism gave me the "out of the box" creativity to find a "better" way of parenting when the training courses provided for foster carers were not helping. I am deeply interested in child and adolescent development. I became involved with Non-Violent Resistance parenting.

> NVR stands for nonviolent resistance. It is an approach that Gandhi and Mandela used during their socio-political movements. It has been developed into a parenting technique by Haim Omer that I believe should be embraced in the whole of parenting, or it can be used simply to focus on "challenging behaviour".
> NVR consists of 9 pillars that work together and stem out of the main core that we call "Parental Presence". NVR is relationship based at its centre. By the parent/carer building strong connection with their child/ren and becoming a firm and secure anchor we see the parent/carer becoming more empowered, positive, safer and stronger in their child/teens life. This produces effective results.

> Parents and carers use these 9 pillars instead of the "behaviour management" parenting techniques (i.e. reward and consequence, time out, etc.).
>
> (Tanner, 2020)

I studied brain development, and emotional intelligence, and was able to put into practice those details which transformed my parenting style. This gave me more understanding of the young people in my care and helped me be fully focused on the child's needs rather than trying to make them fit into something they could not. Foster carers are given "Positive Behaviour" training and expected to use it. However, most of our children will self-sabotage or simply not work with those techniques. So, rather than try and force something that was not working and make the child the problem, I would go on a quest to find something that did work. It would become my special interest and hyper-focus.

My autism enables me to evolve, change, and use different techniques instead of the age-old, "Just do what I do", or even worse, "Just do what I say".

One of my favourite quotes is by Dr Grace Hopper, "The most damaging phrase in the language is. 'it's always been done this way.'" (Hopper, 1987). I quite agree.

My autism makes me very observant. I notice auras and energies, and I can tell when my child is emotional in some way. I can tune into them emotionally without them having to seek me out, when, maybe, they cannot ask for help or explain what is wrong. Does that mean I always understand, agree with, or like the emotions they were feeling? No. But that was for me to vent about with the adults in my support group, including my supervising social worker. It was not up to me to change my child's current state of emotional reality, but to hear it. Many neurotypical parents try to alter their child's present emotional truth and become embroiled in the situation. But I found it more valuable to listen, perhaps because I was used to not being listened to.

My autism makes me very empathetic (not sympathetic!), and my children needed a lot of empathy, grace, and understanding for what they were going through and had been through. Behaviour is communication. It is easy for me to look behind the visible behaviours in a way that is not always easy for neurotypical parents to do. I find neurotypical parents can have a conscious or subconscious love affair with imposed consequences. An imposed consequence is something we put in to control the child's attitude or behaviour and make them stop what they are doing. For example: time out, deprivation of liberties, removal of freedoms or privileges. They may work in the short term but have no long-term effects. The child also can forget they had any accountability and blame shift onto the parent. No child sits in a "time out" contemplating their actions and giving a truthful apology at the end when one is demanded from the parent, "That's your 10 minutes done. Now say sorry and give me a hug". They sit there hating you and obey with the sorry and hug just to get out of time out. No teenager has their iPad removed after being rude to their parents and, while iPadless, sits and considers their attitude problem. They forget their accountability and simply hate you. Imposed consequences do not make them understand their actions. Which is why we have to keep threatening or repeating this method. Also, this method of consequences almost always will escalate any situation. Try keeping that child in a "time out!" Get ready for the backlash and drama when trying to remove something from your teenager.

Among my children, one, who is now a fully-fledged adult, is the star in one of my favourite memories, and they do not mind me retelling it. I think it highlights both how the children may behave because of past trauma and why they may do certain things, and my response and how it would differ from the accepted norm. I had taken this little one to see a matinee of *I Believe in Unicorns* in London. We had a fun train ride, a great theatre trip, and then came back home. They came into the house, got the dustpan and brush out of the cupboard, put them on the kitchen floor, and then absconded. As was the rule, when I could not find them in their usual hiding places, I called the police. They came, found the child, and brought them home. The police explained that the child had said they had absconded as I had made them clean all day! Of course, I had not moved the dustpan and brush as I had not thought about it, so there was the dustpan proof. In front of the officers, I asked the child to take whatever was in their pocket out and hand it to the police. The child, eventually, begrudgingly, did. There were the train and theatre tickets from our trip dated for that day!

For some parents, this would be seen as "naughty behaviour", or worse, and needing a consequence at the very least. After all, the police had been involved and that is always uncomfortable for foster carers. However, I saw it as a child who had had a good time, which was an unknown feeling at this point for them. Having a good time did not feel safe for them, and even though they liked me, liking me felt like a betrayal of their biological parents. It did not need a consequence, it needed empathy. That was something I was able to give. There was nothing more than the natural consequence of being found out. The situation was over, but lessons were learned on all sides that day.

I hear from nearly all my neurotypical parents that they fear the judgement of others. I have no ability to consider this.

My autism meant that, many times, I was able to do things other parents could not because I had no consideration that someone might judge my choices. For example, one of my younger ones had what I still affectionately call "shoe gate" every day. They just hated shoes, and this could, and regularly did, turn into rows. I did not like this as I would rather keep connection with the child, and arguing on a daily basis did not help build our relationship. So, one morning, I let them go to school without any shoes on. (The shoes were in their bag for when they got to school.) They walked barefoot from the car park, through the school playground, and into school. I did not give it a thought. I told friends I had finally ended "shoe gate" and we had had a better morning, and they were horrified. "But what did the other parents think?", I was asked. It had not crossed my mind that other parents in the playground had enough time on their hands to watch me walk my child through that school playground in bare feet. Also, in my head I thought what business was it of theirs?

But I learned two things from this. First, the child found a natural consequence, walking without shoes was uncomfortable, and that changed their attitude to shoes. Secondly, I realised that many neurotypical parents would attempt to make their child conform, and have the constant, draining rows, simply so other parents did not form judgements on them. To me this was madness. Having arguments with your child and making them conform in things which were not important simply for strangers' approval was unnecessary. Equally it did not stop anyone from being judged.

I knew I had experienced "difference" and discrimination throughout my life, so I could relate to my children when they hurt because of those things. Many times, my children would come down at night. At night everything is quiet, it is dark, and a child's mind has space to think about the painful things. Neurotypical parents can get frustrated with this. As we see in a later chapter even a social service manager believed that "once in bed, it's bed". I was able to give half an hour so the child could share their troubles and pass the worry onto someone else, because I understood how frightening nighttime can be.

My autism meant that bluntness and directness, and my refusal to justify myself, helped many an argument with a teenager end more quickly than it would necessarily have done in a neurotypical household! Teenagers will dysregulate and they say cruel things. I learned that neurotypical parents are more likely to respond emotionally to what is being said, therefore elongating the argument. For example:

Teen: You're the worst mum ever.

Mum: How dare you? Do you want me to list everything I do for you?

You can bet the teenager and Mum will get into an unnecessary argument and escalation now.

With me the conversation is more likely to go:

Teen: You're the worst foster carer ever.

Me: Thanks!

Or, if my teenagers said mean things to me, I would generally reply, "Err, rude!" and carry on my life watching *Grey's Anatomy*, or whatever, till they calmed down, when I could then discuss the underlying issue. In the heat of the moment I did not need to justify or explain or validate myself and answer what was really just a series of angry sentences to provoke or continue an argument. I was able to allow a dysregulated teenager time without getting emotionally pulled in, dysregulated myself, or ending up in conflict with them.

Finally, my autism gives me the ability to think of on-the-spot ways to solve potential dramas, which I find hilarious. I have a quick sense of humour. After breakfast one day my child told me they were going on hunger strike – forever! This was in protest at having to eat cereal, toast, or porridge instead of sweets for breakfast. Seemed fair to me! I appreciated their stand. If I had been verbally on this with a "Don't be silly!" or "That's not OK!", it was clear anything I said would be used to create an argument. So, I told them I appreciated their stand, got the calendar and marked off 40 days. I then replied, "No problem. Jesus did 40 days without food. I'll come back to you on 13 March and I will then have to step in and get you to eat. I'm sorry as it might disrupt your hunger strike but let's face that in 40 days!"

This child maintained their hunger strike for two hours till morning snack time! This was always going to have happened. The child was clearly going to want food and in two hours they had forgotten all about their protest. My "humorous" (for me) way of dealing with the situation avoided an "in the moment" drama.

An older teenager decided they were not coming home one night but were going to sleep in a tree in the park. They rang me to tell me their decision. If I had reacted with, "No. You will be in by curfew or else!", there would have been an escalation. They were betting on that happening. The teenager clearly wanted an argument. So, knowing the teenager well, I got a blanket, went to the tree they were in, threw it up so they would not get cold, and asked them to take care as if they fell asleep and fell out of the tree there might be a bump! "See you in the morning", I said and then I went home. The teenager was back pretty soon after, and before curfew. I have many drama-avoiding anecdotes. My sense of humour defused many possible dramas, thankfully!

Cognitive strengths

Auticon's website states:

> Some cognitive strengths tend to be more prevalent in the autism community:
>
> - distinctive logical and analytical abilities
> - sustained concentration and perseverance even when tasks are repetitive
> - conscientiousness, loyalty, and sincerity
> - an exceptional eye for detail and potential errors
> - thorough target versus actual comparisons, and a genuine awareness for quality
> - a strong interest in factual matters and comprehensive technical expertise
>
> (Auticon, 2023)

These things are so important in fostering. Let's look at the plus side of our cognitive strengths:

1. To be able to be logical and analytical over behavioural challenges with our children and teenagers is incredibly important for a foster carer. This means we tend to be able to cope with a lot and not get as stressed or reactive with our children as a neurotypical may. Also, considering we have so many meetings of various kinds, being logical and analytical means that fact and truth are in these meetings. This should be a given but, in my experience, as long as the neurotypical professional delivers their point unemotionally, and with authority, no logic or analytical fact or truth is needed. For example, in one meeting I explained that I had a list that the child's Dr and I had prepared of reasons why we felt this child needed an autism assessment. I read the list out. One professional replied that the child had not displayed any of those characteristics to them. They concluded that the issues were 'due to their diet'. It should be noted that this professional saw the child for less than one hour per week over a very short time frame and I had lived 24/7 with them for several years. I was shocked and asked whether they were "kidding me"! I was then informed that this linked professional had more experience of autism than I did. (Ironic!) There was clearly no logical or analytical thought behind their decision that any issues the child may have were due to diet. No acceptance of the medical backup for the need for an assessment. I was the only one bringing logical and analytical thought to this situation. However, because this professional had a specific degree, a low tone of voice, and an air of authority it was decided by the other professionals in the meeting that these numerous,

obviously autistic, traits were, as had been said, due to diet. The assessment did not happen. To be fair, on this occasion, my "concern" was added into the minutes. However, the outcome remained that "diet" was the cause of all of the issues, hence no assessment was necessary.

2. Sustained perseverance means we will tend not to call time on a placement. This is a big problem in fostering. Foster carers cannot always persevere under the level of stress a child can bring into their home, or when they realise the lack of freedom they will have when fostering a child or young person. So, in many cases, they do call time. Autistic foster carers are highly unlikely to do that. I had three years of serious "child on parent violence". Although I was attacked daily, and lived with screaming tantrums that could last for five hours, I never called time. This was child trauma and I understood it.

3. Conscientiousness, loyalty, and sincerity should be exactly what is desired in a foster carer, and, by nature, autistic foster carers generally show all of these things. These should be the basic building blocks of a system used to care for vulnerable children and young people, on everyone's part.

4. An exceptional eye for detail and potential errors is very useful within fostering. We tend to be able to quicky assess if things will or will not work and, therefore, save a lot of time and potential upset for the children in our care. Many times, in LAC (Looked After Children) meetings, ideas for behaviour management would come up and very quickly I could see, knowing the child in question, whether the ideas would work. Or, more often, if they certainly would not. I would not want to waste time with an idea if I knew it was not going to work. I would ask for more opportunities to

brainstorm so we did not waste our effort on a dead idea. Sometimes I would be told, "No, this is what we do, so let's do it", even if "what we do" would not work with my child. However, I could not back down and agree to trial actions which had no chance of working. Especially not when the next LAC review would not be for another six months, hence wasting half a year on an unhelpful solution for the child. I would be tenacious, always looking for a new idea to prevent potential errors of judgement. Then there is the point of having an exceptional eye for detail which means we notice the smallest change in our children. Maybe it is a tiny eye squint, or a little scratch of the neck, and we know there is a problem. There were many times when I could sense my children were uncomfortable only to be told by a professional without this lived experience, "No they are fine", probably because the signal was so small the professional did not even recognise it. Then the child would go on to have a breakdown because they had been uncomfortable with the situation as I had sensed.

5. When we see that something really does work and is transferable, that is, a deep understanding of brain development, or fostering the NVR parenting way, we can often produce a greater depth of care for our foster children as we tend to be able to adapt ourselves in the pursuit of "quality". Neurodivergents, to a successful or unsuccessful degree, spend every day trying to adapt to a neurotypical majority. It is generally easier for the autistic brain to make big adaptations in both what they do and how they do things than it is for a neurotypical brain. We do not tend to stick with the status quo, especially when it has been seen

not to work on numerous occasions. We look for better alternatives.

6. Let's be honest, if the system wants facts and truth, then they will definitely get them from autistic foster carers. We do tend to "say it as it is" – even when we perhaps should be more circumspect.

I have gone through so much with my children and teenagers over the years. There have been days I am incredibly proud of and days I am seriously not proud of. Many of my children and teenagers are now out of the system and still in regular contact. This proves to me that I parented well and being autistic was not an issue for them. Autistic foster carers are a huge asset to fostering. We may be avant-garde in our parenting style but the children and teenagers we look after probably need a bit of that, if I am being honest. We are loyal, tenacious, persistent. We do not quit when we believe that what we are doing is important. These attributes are needed in foster carers as, too often, foster carers call time when it gets hard. And it does get hard for all of us. However, we need to keep in mind how hard it is for those in our care. They need tenacious advocates to take their corner and fight for their rights and this is something autistic foster carers tend to be very good at.

2
Perceptual differences

Attitude problem

In 2022 I cannot for the life of me remember what the child social worker had said but it rattled my then teenager enough for them to emphatically say, "Megan is autistic". While I felt so proud of them for standing up to power, I was brought down from my proud cloud by the child social worker responding, "Ahh! I knew there was something wrong with her". I was there, she said that to my teenager, and in front of my face.

This gave me two options. (1) Call it out – but, if I did this, I had learned there would be a backlash and I would be labelled as having an attitude problem. Or (2) I could laugh and quip back, at my own expense, to be seen by social services as not having an attitude problem but accepting the low status they afforded me.

I can do both options very well. I can call it out easily and I am able to put myself down to hide my hurt easily too.

Dramatic, uncooperative, rude, argumentative, intense, attitude problem – all these words have been used at various times to describe me. I could never get it right. I could not fit in with social services.

Autistic people can be misunderstood and misrepresented. Social communication and social interaction are different for us. Over the years I have seen all these scattered over Google. Here is a list, not a full list, of examples. I tick every one of them:

1. We can be forthright and direct.
2. We can have high levels of honesty and call out untruths or false information.
3. We can struggle with hiding our thoughts or emotions.
4. We may need to know a satisfactory "why" of what we are told to do or be unable to do it.
5. We may need more clarification than expected.
6. We can be pedantic, very focused on what is right, or questioning nonsensical rules.
7. We can find it hard to let go and can become fixated.
8. We may not understand certain speech patterns. If someone makes a statement we will probably reply with a yes or no and not understand they were hinting for us to actually do something,
9. We may mask or perform in social situations which can appear awkward.
10. We may find eye contact painful.
11. We may have different mannerisms.
12. We may have a flat or heightened tone of voice.

If these traits are seen as part of a person's make up, then they can also be seen as gifts and positives. There may be reasonable adjustments to make if issues come up relating to one of them.

However, if these traits are seen as rude, insubordinate, etc., then this can, and often does, become a character assassination.

Masking

This concept means that I try to change my authentic self in an attempt to fit in. I will try to copy others, or make rules I can follow, so I cannot be seen as contrary or make others uncomfortable.

I mask by a set of rules I have taught myself from watching others. Here are my rules. They run through my head throughout a meeting. I am listening to the meeting but also making sure I have not stopped following these rules:

- smile and laugh a lot;
- make sure I say all the rehearsed polite sentences that need to be said;
- lean forward;
- tilt my head to one side;
- keep my eyes wide and open;
- look people in their eye when they are speaking;
- nod my head continuously when someone is talking;
- put fingers on my lips to stop me talking if an untruth has been said and I need to correct it;
- make sure I start any option I say with, "maybe, perhaps, I'm not sure but", as this makes me sound less direct and abrupt;
- above all, be self-deprecating.

I try to play the part so well, but I come across as an over-exaggerated caricature – so then get labelled as weird or flamboyant.

Sometimes, if I get tired and forget to mask in the meeting, a supervising social worker or child social worker will generally say, "Megan you look confused". They would be right. They mean I have stopped masking, so I have my "normal" face on and it does look blank or confused.

The amount of effort it takes to keep masking normally means that if, in a meeting, a trigger is pushed, I instantly drop the mask and from sheer exhaustion I end up either crying in frustration, walking out, or speaking my frank and very truthful mind. Which, after appearing like the happiest clown alive, is an extraordinary nanosecond flip and again leads to labels of being rude, dramatic, intense, and uncooperative.

Masking is unsustainable for me. I have never been good at it and the impacts of trying to mask are anxiety, self-hatred, chronic stress, and depression – both for me and most autistics.

Afterwards I will play the meeting over and over in my head, over-analysing every moment of it and feeling that social workers are justified in their assessment of my character and personality.

Different initial premises

During the Form F interview, which is the process you go through to become a foster carer, my fridge was examined, and I was told there was no fridge thermometer and I needed to get one.

I felt that was silly and asked, "Really?!" My assessor explained that it was a requirement and they needed to tick that I had a fridge thermometer in place before I could pass the Form F.

I was surprised that this was serious. I had obviously misunderstood the importance and I wanted to be able to have the same understanding as my assessor. Considering the fridge had a temperature dial and was on the correct setting I asked for help to understand the reasoning behind this.

- What does the thermometer show me that I do not already know?
- Does a fridge's temperature fluctuate? If so, I didn't know that.
- Do I need to look at the thermometer at certain times of the day?
- Who would I call if the thermometer gave an unsatisfactory reading?
- Do you need a daily/weekly spreadsheet of the readings?

My assessor saw my questions as being rude and cocky. I was confused. Initially when I asked her if she was really serious I guess I was being rude by not accepting her knowledge and authority, but once she had explained the necessity of a fridge thermometer to becoming a foster carer, I was all in.

My curiosity, understanding, need for clarification, and interest levels were high, and I was willing to learn and change my view from "this is stupid" to "this is important".

The problem with this is, it was stupid! No one ever looked at my fridge thermometer or brought it up again. Once I passed the Form F it was forgotten, it just sat there in the fridge, and I was none the wiser as to why.

The assessor must have known this and assumed I must know it too, which is why she took my questions as rude. She thought I must know it was pointless, but I just needed to get one. I thought, "Wow, I never knew this. Interesting. I want to know all about it".

We were looking at the situation from two different perspectives. My autistic intrigue came across as sarcasm.

Attempting to understand

I am hyper-focused on trying to understand, being able to conform and say or do the right thing. The success rate is not high, because my brain cannot think the way a neurotypical's does.

Some autistic people are unable to work out facial or body language. I went to drama college so had a good three years of learning how people use their face and body for communication.

I have made lists, found patterns, created rules focusing on facial and body language which help me see if the spoken words are what they mean.

I need to hear words and to see the body or facial language when I am in a meeting. Meetings changed during Covid from face to face to being over Teams. I noticed that cameras did not have to be on for the professionals in the meetings.

Now, some autistic people like this, but for me I need to see faces; preferably the whole person, but, if not that, then the face at least. In my general life I cannot use the telephone or listen to voicemails as simply a voice can hide so much.

Neurotypical people often say words which disagree with their truth. If I cannot see the person, it is not easy for me to know what their words mean.

A simple example. I may come into a meeting and ask, "How are you?" The child social worker says, "Fine". They may be fine or they may not be fine and the only way I can tell is via their facial indicators. Neurotypical people will generally say "fine" regardless of whether it is true or not. However, their face could be showing that they are actually furious or sad.

That is a simple example, but if we go further along the lines of words and facial expression or body language not matching up I am going to misunderstand conversations if I only have the words given to me.

If I misunderstand conversations I can come across as disinterested, unempathetic, or short, when the reality is that I took the words as fact, but was expected to "read between the lines", or understand that what someone says and what someone thinks are not always in agreement.

I remember a linked professional (please refer to the Glossary) calling me one day and in a very calm, kind voice saying down the phone, "Do you think you can use a reward chart in your home?" I replied in a very friendly and happy way, "No". (Reward charts are not helpful for a lot of children for well-documented reasons.) The linked professional tried again, "You don't think it would be a good idea?" I replied, again, in a very friendly and kind way, "No". I felt the conversation went well. She was questioning an idea she had had, and I helped her by saying that it was not going to work.

However, based on that conversation, I was labelled as uncooperative with professionals. But, as autistic people, we speak directly to the words spoken to us. If someone wants to give us a directive it needs to be a directive, not said as a question. I was not asked why "no" was my opinion, so I did not give a "why". I did not know it was an issue, or necessary. In my head the linked professional was just "wondering" through ideas with me, asking questions which had yes or no answers. In her head she was giving me a directive. One of the most frustrating things I find is when I ask someone a question requiring a yes or no answer and I get the answer plus "because …" and a whole stream of words I do not need. I am forever saying, "If I needed a because, or a why, I would ask for it". Neurotypicals always seem to need to justify their "yes" or "no" with a "because" monologue. This is another reason why an autistic person can appear "short".

Predetermined expectations

I may not respond in a way that aligns with a social worker's expectation.

Sitting in the "Journey to Foster" meetings, the three-day course potential foster carers go on, the social worker handed us an A4 sheet with boxes on it and in the boxes were words like toys, clothes, friends, siblings, parents, favourite foods. "When a child comes into care, they lose everything. I am going to read each of these boxes out and when I do you need to cross them out on your sheet and see how you feel."

During the exercise I could hear from other potential carers comments of, "Oh gosh. I feel so sad. This hurts". The social worker then asked us, individually, to share how we felt. Everyone there was very emotionally affected by it. I was confused. I was not looking forward to my turn. When asked I said, "I feel nothing because the exercise isn't real. I can empathise for the children and how they must feel but crossing out words on a sheet isn't the same and I don't feel anything".

I clearly remember everyone looking at me with a surprised expression. The social worker went on to ask: "Ok. What would you do if this happened to you?" Everyone replied along the lines of, "I'd cry. I'd need love, care, attention. I'd close down. I'd be so hurt inside I'd need someone to open me up again with love". My turn: "I'd pay you back for taking everything away from me".

This was not the correct answer. Everyone laughed nervously and the social worker said how thankful she was that I was not the child for the sake of whoever my social worker would be.

Their correct answer was that the child would be so sad and need love. However, I must say that, after fostering three children and nine teenagers, I have learned that my answer was far more realistic than the expected and desired answer was!

Looking back, the social worker had primed us for the expected response in the way she phrased the activity, but at the time I had not learned how to read the room and answer in agreement, even if it was not my truth.

I did not understand that there was a predetermined expectation of what the answer should be. Everyone seemed to know that but me. I did not understand that it was not a genuine request for my opinion. I was laughed at and put down and felt confused. I had not "got it". I had misunderstood the communication. This was on the first few days of my fostering journey, and it would be a constant throughout my time as a foster carer.

Another example of predetermined expectation can be something as simple as just sitting. There is a natural expectation that we sit on a chair, feet on the floor, hand in lap, or arms crossed. It is expected. We are taught this at school. It is normal. It is how it is done. However, @theautisticlife says: "Proprioception is the sense that provides information to our brains about where our body is in space. Autistic people often have proprioceptive differences due to our sensory processing systems and, as a result, may have a hard time sitting still or in 'typical' ways" (The Autistic Life, 2021).

If I sit on a chair in the "normal" way my brain does not get enough proprioceptive input so my body physically ends up hurting. It is so uncomfortable that I will fidget or need to get up. I stop concentrating on what I need to be focusing on because I am overwhelmed with how my body is feeling. I normally sit on a chair with one leg up with one foot on the chair seat, or I sit sideways in a chair with my legs hanging over the chair arm. Sometimes I sit with one leg under me on the chair, but I will probably change position often, especially during a long conversation or meeting. When I cannot sit like this I will get up and go to the bathroom regularly, not because I need the toilet, but it gives an acceptable excuse to get up when I need to move to relax my hurting body.

I was in a meeting once, I seem to remember it was a PEP meeting, so teachers, social workers, CAMHS, and myself were present. I was subconsciously moving in my chair trying to keep focus and look presentable while sitting, making as little fuss as I could. Slow, gentle shifts I have found over the years can go unnoticed or at least they are generally unmentioned. However, in this meeting someone asked, "Are you ok? Can I ask you to sit still please?" I felt so humiliated. For the rest of the meeting I tried my hardest to be still, and I think I achieved it, but I cannot remember anything else of importance about that meeting even though I have a very clear memory of facts that happened over the years, as this book shows! All my focus was taken up achieving the expectation that I could sit on this chair for one and a half hours perfectly still. If I had been able to move, or get up, or stand against the wall, I would have had full focus on the meeting as my body would not have hurt the way it did.

When autistics move or shift positions it gives our brain the messages from our muscles and joints to know where our body parts are in relation to each other. There is a physical reason why we autistics cannot sit "normally", in a way which is classed as being "acceptable".

I also, even as an adult, slump at a desk. I put my elbows on the table. I would rather sit than run or jump as I am clumsy and can trip over air. I have difficulty with fine motor tasks. All of these are to do with me having an under-responsive proprioceptive input.

On a humorous aside, the difficulty with fine motor tasks can get you into serious trouble with adults, or, if you are with children, you can end up really laughing.

My first foster child was a mid-aged teenager so this issue did not come up with them, but then I had a little 8-year-old. In my attempt at trying to be that fun, energised, excitable foster mum I would give a countdown of 3, using my fingers to start something. Unfortunately, it would always end up with me giving a naughty middle finger salute. I was utterly incapable of working out how to face my hand and count my fingers down in a different way. We would end up really laughing and it became my little one's favourite part of any games. "Do the 3 countdown Megan" they would shout. "Yeah, that's a no because I know why you want that! LOL". I had to ask this little 8-year-old foster child how to use my fingers to countdown from 3 without me making the flip sign. We laughed a lot at that one. But they helped me turn my hand the right way round and count my fingers down politely. It was no longer so funny for them after I had learned a more appropriate way. Needless to say, they did not want the 3 countdown anymore!

They never told their social worker this story, but I often wonder what would have happened if they had, what their reaction would have been. Because of my prolonged experiences, I am sure it would not have been seen as humorous! I am sure it would, in fact, have been a problem.

I could easily see this story being reframed and written in a report as, "Megan has used an inappropriate middle finger sign to the child five times this past month. It got to the point where the child had to correct Megan".

And this brings up a very good point. It is sad that in my head I think this. It is sad that I worry about everything and how it can be misconstrued and misrepresented. And it is sad that I 100 per cent believe that most stories will be taken with a "dark side" first until the light in them is proven, and even then the positive side will probably not be believed.

Can autistics have a sense of humour?

This is the same as for neurotypicals; some do and some do not. Yet, in my case, yes, I find myself hilarious. Many times, people have said to me that they find the way I phrase things, do things, or my perception of things incredibly funny. They are right. I can laugh at myself, and at others, and I do see things from an amusing perspective. To be fair, we autistics need something to create balance in life or we would all be hiding under the bed sheets forever!

One person congratulated me on writing this book. I wrote back with, "If you find I have disappeared, my new name is Heidi and I'm living in Austria!)" She replied, "Only you can turn a broken system into a heartfelt and amusing adventure highlighting the seriousness of the issue with your honest experiences. Best of luck. Kx"

I posted on Facebook making fun of my pet rabbit, who is a badly behaved creature if ever I knew one. A friend replied. "Is it your autism that causes you to put a hilarious twist on everything – or just your natural comic genius? They might be one and the same thing!"

My children and young people loved my humour. It is often unapologetically naughty, so children and teenagers definitely appreciate it. However, as we see in the introduction, if I am using humour to defuse an issue, it might not be as funny for them. Then, it is probably best for them to jump on that gravy train and use the humorous answer I give them as their "get out" clause.

My humour can also be inappropriate. I probably would not find funny what you find funny. I am not great at "social interaction" humour, so I may come across as not having a sense of humour at all. I just do not get it. But I will find people funny, maybe not for the right reasons! I am not good with contrived forms of humour. I will not "get the joke".

Hannah Gadsby, an autistic comedian, says, "To give you an idea of what it feels to be on the spectrum, basically what it feels like is being the only sober person in a room full of drunks or the other way round. Basically, everyone is operating on a wavelength you can't quite key in to. I never get the memo, I never do" (Gadsby, 2020).

I am howling while writing that quote – now that is my humour!

Echolalia

"A large number of people with autism, about 75 per cent, experience echolalia" (Rudy, 2022). Echolalia is when we repeat words or phrases. I do this when I am anxious, unsure, confused, or heading into overwhelm. I may repeat the question I am asked or a phrase that has been said. Or, when I have completed a task I have been given, I will praise myself. I also speak in quotes, especially if I am trying to get heard. I will repeat relevant quotes from various pieces of research to reinforce what I mean. In emails to social workers, to try and get my point across, I will often use quotes from a variety of people, including Brene Brown to Shakespeare!

Reasonable adjustments

1. Understand we are not rude, obnoxious, dramatic, impertinent, obtuse. We see things differently and express things differently.
2. If we are asking too many questions, it is because we need heightened levels of understanding to be able to accomplish tasks. So be patient and let us ask our questions to gain understanding.

3. Do not assume we understand your premise. You may see a 9 but we may see a 6!
4. Do not pose demands as questions: "Would you like to join the meeting?" may get a "No thank you", response and nonattendance. If we are needed, state it. "Please come to the meeting at 10 a.m."
5. Understanding echolalia will help social workers to not take offence or feel that we are being obtuse. For us it is normal.
6. Do not expect eye contact. Eye contact is painful. I have trained myself to make eye contact when someone is speaking to me but I am unable to give eye contact when I am speaking. This is not rudeness.
7. Allow stimming. I play with Blu Tack or a hairband. Another autistic may do different things. This helps us. We are not ignoring you. In fact, it is the opposite, it helps us focus.
8. Remember our muscles, joints, and tendons can require different activities to yours and we may need to move more or less than you would. So let us stand, walk around at the back of room, or even sit on the floor. This way we will not disturb anyone visually but can focus better than when we are expected to sit properly, be in pain, and, therefore, not pay attention.
9. If there have to be games involving throwing or other activities that require fine motor skills as an ice breaker in training sessions or meetings we may want to be excused. We may not have the same fine motor skills ability that every other adult in the room has and it is humiliating.
10. If you feel we are being judgemental, ask us. We will probably not realise we are distressing or annoying you.

If we do realise, we will not know why or how to sort it in a way that is best for you and your needs. If you are able to directly ask, "Are you being intentionally uncooperative/rude/argumentative?", we are then able to explain, "Gosh, no. I simply do not understand but am trying my best. I am feeling confused and I need help with 'xyz'".

These reasonable adjustments do not take time or effort or large financial costs. They simply revolve around challenging your assumptions, appreciating difference, and being non-judgemental and inclusive.

Autistic people are highly sensitive, so the last thing we are trying to do is to be one of these negative labels or judgements. If you think an autistic foster carer is being unhelpful it is much kinder to assume there is miscommunication and that we are not being difficult or have an attitude problem. We really are doing our very best.

3
Executive functioning differences

What is executive functioning?

Executive function: the group of complex mental processes and cognitive abilities (such as working memory, impulse inhibition, and reasoning) that control the skills (such as organizing tasks, remembering details, managing time, and solving problems) required for goal-directed behavior.

(Merriam-Webster Dictionary, 2023)

Executive functions (EFs) make possible mentally playing with ideas; taking the time to think before acting; meeting novel, unanticipated challenges; resisting temptations; and staying focused. Core EFs are inhibition [response inhibition (self-control – resisting temptations and resisting acting impulsively) and interference control (selective attention and cognitive inhibition)], working memory, and cognitive flexibility (including creatively thinking "outside the box," seeing anything from different perspectives, and quickly and flexibly adapting to changed circumstances).

(Diamond, 2013)

Some sources say that up to 80% of those with autism suffer from executive function disorder, leading to difficulties managing time, completing tasks, and making what for many of us would be simple tasks – like cleaning our rooms – very complicated or seemingly impossible.

The technical definition of executive function is: the cognitive processes that help us regulate, control and manage our thoughts and actions. It includes planning, working memory, attention, problem solving, verbal reasoning, inhibition, cognitive flexibility, initiation of actions and monitoring of actions.

(Bennie, 2018)

Eighty per cent of autistic people! That is the majority. So it is more than likely that an autistic foster carer will struggle with aspects of executive functioning.

From a personal point of view, I can easily think "outside the box". Most of what I do or come up with is "outside the box". I am also a solution-based thinker so problem solving comes easily to me. Unless I am under pressure, then I blank and freeze.

I have learned to make my environment relaxed and pressure-less. This way I can work easily at my optimum. However, when working with social services I am not able to control my environment. Social workers often introduce pressure or stress into my environment, either consciously or subconsciously, and

I have no control over that. This can affect my ability to process, react, or respond.

You might consider that children or teenagers obviously bring their pressures or stress into any environment. But that is to be expected, they are children. We have our support group to go to if we need to let off steam. I can handle that and work with it. It is when adults transfer stress or pressure that I am not able to respond quickly, especially when it comes out of the blue.

I struggle with the following aspects.

Working memory

The prefrontal cortex is where working memory lives. The autistic prefrontal cortex can have around 67 per cent more neurons compared to a non-autistic person (Courchesne and Pierce, 2005). When an autistic person is asked to remember or process information there is less activity in the prefrontal cortex than there is in a neurotypical brain (Koshino et al., 2005). "Furthermore, when a child with ASD [autism spectrum disorder] is presented with two tasks and has to focus on one while ignoring the other distracting task, their brain activity reveals that they do not actually shift their attention to the more important information" (Luna et al., 2002).

I cannot hold onto information that is not important. What is important to me may not be what is important to someone else, and vice versa. I fostered many children and teenagers with serious trauma who would abscond for a variety of reasons. When this happens, you have to call the police. The police go through a questionnaire and within this you are asked seemingly simple questions, such as "What is the child wearing?", or "What hairstyle does the young person have today?" I would not be able to remember these things. Even if I had personally put the child's hair into plaits in the morning, later in the day I would not know what I had done with their hair. A child could have a pair of trainers I had bought them six months ago, usually after long discussions, but I would have no clue what colour they were.

Another example of this is when your supervising social worker comes over and asks you very simple or mundane questions, for example: "What did Kim have for breakfast?". Although I would have made breakfast, and been there while it was eaten, I would not have a clue what it consisted of once the meal was over.

If things are not important at the moment of execution, my brain does not retain the information. As you can imagine this can look very bad if a social worker or professional is asking questions on very simple things and I have no idea of the answers. Ask me something of importance and I will always be able to answer, with every small detail included.

Planning and organisation

Nothing will get done unless I have a list. If something is suddenly sprung on me, adding it in or making changes in order to be able to do it is a big problem. A social worker may send an email saying, "Can you send me a copy of the child's passport by lunch". To do this, first, I need to find a space in the few hours before the deadline to align my focus for this unexpected task, then make a space to achieve it (which is another issue involving even more steps as I then have to reschedule the rest of my morning list). Then I have to work out where it is, and find it, and scan it, and send it to them. That is a lot of planning to fulfil the simple request they have asked me to achieve by lunchtime. This may seem a simple thing to most people but, for people who struggle with executive functioning, it can be nigh on impossible. Every day is planned out in full the night before so I can make sure I achieve all I need to achieve within the given time constraints. Surprises with a limited timeframe for delivery can be extremely difficult and I can freeze so that I just do not get it done. I have whiteboards all over the kitchen for this very reason and every one of my children know that if they tell me anything of importance, they need to write it on the whiteboard too. That way it will be added into the plans. It works.

Staying focused

I cannot sit still and pay attention. For example, supervision is so difficult because your supervising social worker comes to your house and for one and a half to two hours you sit and talk. Most of what you talk about is information which has already been spoken of or emailed, so it is repetition. Although autistic people may repeat intense interests and certain repetitive behaviours as a source of enjoyment and a way of coping with everyday life, these conversations probably do not fall into that category for us. During this meeting there is a lot of small talk or superficial waffle because it is "polite". Unfortunately, my attention has run out in 20 minutes and the rest of the time is mentally exhausting. This difficulty makes us look rude and disinterested. We are not. When I was with the fostering agency I was lucky enough to have the same supervising social worker for the whole time. I respected and liked her a lot. However, I still could not sit and talk about things for one and a half to two hours. I would be clock watching and waning fast. We are quick off the mark. A good solid 20 minutes talking about anything that has not been already said is better than two hours of time wasting. My friends will tell you I am exactly the same with them!

Impulse inhibition

> Inhibitory control, also known as response inhibition, is a cognitive process and one facet of executive function that permits an individual to inhibit their impulses and natural, habitual, or dominant behavioral responses to stimuli (i.e., learned prepotent responses) in order to select more appropriate behaviors that are consistent with one's goals.
>
> (Li et al., 2022)

This can look like:

- interrupting conversations;
- having trouble taking turns;
- having angry outbursts;
- being easily distracted and having trouble paying attention;
- having trouble remembering and following instructions;
- blurting out answers before being called on or before the question is finished.

I struggle with all of this a lot when working alongside adults. I often fall into impulse inhibition behaviours, a bit like a teenager. Before I have time to think I have said what you cannot say or rolled my eyes or interrupted. If there is a lot of waffle I will lose attention, or just speak without waiting my turn, to speed things up. If I am not being heard, or if I seem to be deliberately misunderstood or misrepresented, and I cannot make it better, I will show anger and cry. If someone says something that shocks me my face will show it. I am not able to deliver a "more appropriate behaviour" if it is inconsistent with my truth or, frankly, the truth.

I remember a few training sessions which were on subjects I knew a lot about so the training was easy. The facilitator would ask questions and immediately I would blurt out the answer, not even thinking to let someone else have a go. I did not even realise I was doing it. Sometimes the facilitator had to say, "Someone other than Megan". I probably came across as rather annoying. However, this is impulse inhibition pure and simple. The question was asked, I knew the answer, it came right out of my mouth.

For me impulse inhibition can be clearly seen in such situations, but for others it may show up if sensory overload is happening. When I am feeling sensory overload it can lead to impulse inhibition behaviours, but I am normally able to excuse myself from the environment or ask for changes to help ease the sensory issues which are affecting me. It is harder for me to remove myself or ask for changes in conversations which is why conversations are my biggest issue. This is when impulse inhibition comes to the fore for me.

Time management

Some autistic people struggle because of difficulty tracking and managing time. Some operate on a very loose schedule, unaware of what time it is and how long it may take to accomplish a task. Others adhere very rigidly to a schedule – sometimes managing a schedule minute to minute.

(CAR Autism Roadmap, 2020)

Time does not have much meaning for me. Although I have an amazing memory for details of conversations, I do not remember if things happened yesterday or two weeks ago. I do not remember dates or times. This can cause problems if your social worker is asking what time "xyz" happened. It is a given that everyone must know what day or time things occurred. Unfortunately, autistics really may not be able to remember. I can start an action and not know if it will require a short or long timeframe to finish it. Equally, I can say, "Yes, I will do that now", but now may mean in three weeks' time. I have a diary that I plan everything for the day in and a running to-do list. When I am in a safe space, I may not stick rigidly to it. But the more overwhelmed I get, the more rigid I become with my diary and to-do list.

Yes, we may have struggles with executive functioning, but there are also many cognitive strengths which we can bring to the table (see Chapter 1).

Reasonable adjustments

1. **Working memory**: Remember that we may not remember things easily. If we do not remember what we made our child for dinner last night it does not mean the child did not eat, nor are we being obtuse. If you want us to do something important keep it simple and straight. Do not add any, "Oh, also"s. The best way to ensure we complete new tasks would be to write an email and simply bullet point the list of what you would like rather than tell us verbally.

2. **Planning and organisation**: We need reminders and deadlines. If logs or reports are due, they will probably be done at the eleventh hour. Maybe you will receive them past midnight on the due date. So, be flexible when possible, or ensure you give a firm deadline if needed, rather than a "when you can" or "sometime soon can you?" Our answer may be, "No".

3. **Staying focused**: Let us stim, fiddle, or move. You probably will have 100 per cent of our attention when we do this. When we are sitting still and looking as if we are fully involved, we are probably not listening at all.

4. **Impulse inhibition**: If the cause is due to sensory issues, see what changes you can make to the environment. For example, remove room scents like air fresheners, be aware of bright strip lights, turn the noisy air conditioning off for a while. Simple changes can radically reduce sensory overload. If it is communication that can spark impulse inhibition, let the foster carer remove themselves for a while if they are finding conversations difficult. Most meetings are all talk with limited, if any, action. Most meetings have "flexible" truths spoken in them. This is often the way of the system. Unfortunately, autistics cannot cope with this. Let us leave the meeting for a while. If we respond with a less than appropriate answer we will apologise later (probably for how we expressed the response, not actually for what we did or said). There would have been absolute honesty in what we were trying to express. Understand that the communication, at that time, was too much, and we could not or were not allowed to leave, meaning that the situation became overwhelming. Sometimes the truth we say does hurt professionals. They will get a lot of truth from autistic

foster carers. But if they understand it is because we believe the truth holds the helpful answers and solutions then they can also understand that we are coming from a positive place. If the autistic foster carer is known to answer first, call out, or not take turns in training sessions or meetings, and it is not helpful, then remind them beforehand that in this meeting we need to "xyz". They will be thankful for the reminder.

5. **Time management**: Your autistic foster carer should live with diaries and to-do lists. If they do not, encourage them to do this as it will help supervisions, logs, reports, and so much more. If your autistic foster carer cannot remember a time or date which you need, walk them through the period so that you can see what they do remember and go from there. For example, "What day was the child's sports day?" The foster carer cannot remember. Let them look through and check their diaries or to-do lists. Do not expect them to remember without looking. If they cannot find the date, then walk them through their week. "Okay, let's see, Monday was the child's end of term show, Tuesday they had the tummy bug, they finished school on Thursday so could it have been Wednesday?" Anything that can prompt something which aids their memory of the date.

6. Although I am one of the autistics who is able to think outside the box, and this is an attribute for many autistic people as we have seen, there may be some autistic foster carers who do not have this ability. So, be mindful that autism is a spectrum disorder, it is not linear. We are all going to have differing strengths and weaknesses, just as allistics do. ("Allistic" refers to people who are not on the autism spectrum.) If you want creative thinking in a meeting check

first. If needed, then help them, brainstorm with them. Do not expect a brain to do what it cannot do just because your brain can do it without prompts.

When considering executive functioning it is important to remember that we do not think or work the same as neurotypicals and we may express ourselves, focus, or think differently. That does not mean incorrectly. It means it just does not look the same as for you. That is okay. To be okay with "difference" you do actually have to be okay with "difference" and not just have it as a policy, a strap line, or even a verbal affirmation. When our executive functioning differences are presented during meetings or training sessions, this is where we soon see how inclusive social services really are, when our differences are not accepted or respected as of equal worth!

4
Social differences

The social aspect of fostering

Workplace socials are intended to increase happiness, engage employees, connect people, and team build. I can see how some people, especially those who live with a social goal in life, need this. Social services put on lots of events for foster carers, and I do think this is very valuable for most neurotypical carers. I have watched them; they enjoy themselves. So, I certainly am not asking for such events to stop. Just maybe stop making us autistics go along. Here is why.

Autistics generally do not have a social goal in the things we choose to do. To engage with other people, make small talk, give or receive compliments or praise, talk about things that are not our special interest, do whatever is needed to make others happy or show that we are happy from what we are receiving, is exhausting, draining, and anxiety producing. These social events may bring us closer to autistic burnout and chronic stress!

This is because autistics generally care very little for these things. As a foster carer I was child-focused not social-focused. I had a well-chosen support group of my own, handpicked over the years. If I needed a social event, it would be with them.

I loved being a foster carer. Parenting the children and teenagers became a special interest I could absorb myself in. I did it well, very well, and this gave me great satisfaction.

But fostering brings a mountain of social demands. You are not only expected to attend social gatherings, but should participate in, and enjoy, them. Social services wanted to put on events which increased happiness, but for me they had a huge negative impact on my mind and body. The list below did not have the intended results for me:

- Foster carer appreciation events
- Monthly support groups
- WhatsApp groups or Facebook groups
- Training days (I add these because of the four hours they took to complete at least two hours would be spent in socialising, not in training)
- School holiday days out – e.g. Legoland trips (although we acknowledge they are loved by our children or teenagers)
- Christmas events.

Spoon theory

Christine Miserandino came up with the spoon theory when she was trying to explain her chronic illness (Miserandino, 2003). Autistics have taken it on. It means that, whereas most people have more than enough spoons for the day, we only have a certain number of spoons in a day, and, when they are gone, they are gone. Executive functioning, sensory issues, communication, focus and physical demands, for example, all take up spoons. Spoons are like energy units and autistic people do not have as many energy units as neurotypicals.

I was a single carer fostering very traumatised children and teenagers. I was working from home in a self-employed capacity. I had the house to upkeep. I had social services "meaningful appointments" to invest in. I had my family and friends. I had my dog. That is a lot of executive functioning, sensory and communication issues, focus, and physical investments that my limited energy spoons had to be spread out for.

I had to get someone, generally my mother, to come and help with parts of my day so I did not run out of spoons. She would come in the evening and do bits and bobs to ease the load in areas that she could help with, so I could use my spoons for the parts I needed to do.

I had made reasonable adjustments so I could make it work by outsourcing things to someone who had many more spoons and could help. But then throw in the social side, events here, days out there, celebration ceremonies, support group meetings, and the WhatsApp group pinging off! I had no spare spoons for these and I could not always outsource these things to someone who could go in my place!

Social hangover

Autistics call this feeling of depletion a social hangover. We have to mask so much and change the mask depending on the person we are interacting with. We must pretend we are interested in things we are not interested in. We have to navigate all the unspoken rules of engagement.

If you remember an actual hangover, or have experienced something similar, you know the feeling. We can feel physically sick; our body can ache; we can get a headache; we can even be unable to speak for a while. Mentally we can become paranoid, worried, anxious, blank, and overwhelmed. We can get this feeling after any social occasion, not just those related to fostering. For example, my friends will say, "I'm having a big party. I'd love you to come. I know you can't cope, so please don't come. I just want you to know that you are invited with no expectation of arrival". Or recently my best friend said, "So, Megan. Continuing my 40th celebration I'm having a very small gathering at my house and then out to dinner. Hardly anyone for this. You can do it! See you there". My friends tell me whether it will be too much or not because they know me well. Either way the invite is there without expectation if they know it is too much, or with expectation if they know I could cope. They are always "autism focused" not "self-focused".

I know my social hangover is coming on when I become even more hypersensitive than normal and my nervous system kicks in. I go into flight or freeze mode and I can feel that I am going to melt down, cry, or run away.

It can take a day or so to recover from a dinner or social event. To recover means I need to sleep, do something that involves no thinking, or maybe get absorbed in a special interest to pick me back up. If I am fostering a child or teenager, I do not have a day to sleep or sit watching *NCIS* for 36 hours with the curtains closed to reboot.

Sensory aspect

It is worth noting that "recent studies highlighted that autistic individuals show increased perceptual capacity – the ability to process more information at any one time" (Brinkert and Remington, 2020). Autistics can have hypersensitivity or hyposensitivity to sight, sounds, smells, tastes, touch, balance, and body awareness. I am hypersensitive to all the senses.

- **Visual**: bright, fluorescent, or flashing lights, the air particles that fly around, loud colours on room walls or dramatic wallpaper all affect me. Colours move and speak! Maybe the training room for fostering is decked out like a classroom – painted yellow and red and with lots of children's art on it – fussy and exhausting for my eyes.
- **Sound**: the noise of lots of people speaking at once, or music and speaking, hearing electricity, or the buzz of a light, or the wind. My family have a tendency to whisper, whispering physically hurts me. For me even the noise of stroking the dog can hurt. I had to train my children and teenagers how to stroke our dog, so it did not make a painful noise. Unexpected or unpredictable sounds can make me jump or look startled. Doorbells, something ringing, a chair scraping across the floor, cutlery on a plate are all issues.
- **Smells**: the smells from the room, perfumes, bodies, and even the environment. I could smell my teenagers spraying their deodorant from a mile away, and once in my nose I could not get it out. I was able to explain the effect this had on me and we used stick or roll-on deodorants, not sprays, in the house. However, I cannot ask a social worker to wash her perfume off!
- **Touch**: the handshakes, hugs, and air kisses that are expected. People may even brush past us, nothing in itself, but the brush past feels like hot pokers. Maybe we have to wear a certain smart or casual outfit and we have difficulties with

the texture of clothing that works for the event. It is itchy, painful, scratchy, touching in a "wrong" way, e.g. for me it may be too close to my neck, or just t-shirt sleeves that are flapping on my arm intermittently.

I also have vestibular hypersensitivity. I find it hard to walk on uneven surfaces like cobble stones. I lose my balance easily and changing walking direction is difficult.

Our brains receive too much information from given situations and we cannot process it. We are not able to select what we should focus on. Bombardment is a perfect word.

At first, I would attend these events. But trying to concentrate on a conversation someone was having with me while my senses were going crazy was too much, so I opted to stay away.

Small talk

The Cambridge dictionary defines small talk like this: small talk is conversation about things that are not important, often between people who do not know each other well. I cannot do small talk. Apart from being superficial and adding no real value, it is incredibly boring to hear stories from people I do not know or am not interested in.

Small talk exists so people feel connected. People need to feel seen and heard and small talk is a perfect vehicle for this. It is a social goal. You have a non-verbal agreement, or laugh at something which is very inconsequential, and feel bonded by the ritual. I do not need validation in a small talk way.

I cannot connect to someone unless the conversation is interesting. If the content of the conversation is engaging, then

I am more likely to feel connected. Once I realised small talk is not to gain any important knowledge, or to really desire to hear the answers, it became painful. I am now more likely to be monosyllabic, give one-word answers or parrot back words they said to me. This exchange actually happened at a fostering event.

- **Person:** When is your birthday?
- **Me:** 24 June.
- **Person:** Wow. My cousin has the same birthday as you.
- **Me:** Wow. (It is not wow, I do not care, I do not know your cousin, but the person has told me it is a wow, so I know that is what I say – tilt head to side, smile widely, and raise eyebrows.)
- **Person:** Yes, how amazing is that!
- **Me:** Yes, amazing. (Again, I parrot back their words hoping that is the correct answer. Is it amazing though? Really? No, it is not as around 20.8 million people will have the same birthday as me, but keep head tilted and nod lots. Also, I remember I am supposed to ask the question back to them, but I just cannot bring myself to ask. I do not honestly want to know.)

The person felt connected and happy. I felt this was the dumbest interaction of the evening and the bar was low. I liked the person. They were lovely. But the conversation was disappointing. At a fostering social, event or day out no one ever came up to me and said, "Oh, have you heard this new idea to stop animal poaching?", or brought something inspiring or interesting to the conversation. At a social event it was a revolving door of small talk or feigned interest.

Words for information

Because we, as autistic people, use words to genuinely gain information, we believe others do too. If you asked me, "How are you?", before I learned that the answer was "Fine thank you", I would go into depth about my internal emotional state at the time. Ask me, "What are your plans for the weekend?" and settle in for the ride! I will give you the timed plans from waking up and getting showered on Saturday morning to going to bed on Sunday evening. We are literal, we will answer literally. Generally, they are not the answers that are wanted!

Info-dumping

Autistics can also info-dump. If you say to me, "The weather is nice today", I may launch into an answer on how altocumulus clouds really are beautiful and give you some of my cloud facts, because I do love clouds and I thought, because you expressed pleasure at the weather, you liked clouds too!

Gossip

I understand that if you get a group of people together who are all foster carers then gossip will happen. Fostering is hard. Gossip is a vehicle for expressing emotions, letting off steam, gaining and giving validation and group bonding against an issue or another clique.

It also has well documented negative sides! In one foster carer coffee morning a conversation like this took place:

> **Person 1 to Person 2:** "Oh, gosh, have you heard about Alice; I am so concerned about her."

We should be honest here; this is not true concern. It is usually a masked meanness as the next sentence is going to be something that is not positive or praiseworthy. It is not concern. It is the veil through which negative information can be shared about someone else to somebody who really has no right to the information. This may be something along the lines of, "She is really struggling with her foster teen, she's at a loss and it's not the first time. I wonder if she's OK and able to keep going for much longer".

Person 2 clearly does not know there had been a problem, so it probably is not their business. Equally, Alice may not have wanted that information shared even if the information was correct in the first place.

If Person 1 said to me, "Oh, gosh. Have you heard about Alice? I am so concerned about them", I would definitely reply, "No. I've not. If you are concerned, why don't you go and speak to her".

I think that is the kindest answer personally. I do not want Person 1 to talk about someone behind their back. But I would happily bet you that Person 1 will not think of it as a kind or caring answer as their desire to gossip has been thwarted! All too often they would then search out Person 3 and say something along the lines of, "I tried to tell Megan about Alice and she shut me down. She didn't care or want to hear. She really doesn't have empathy, does she?"

I have written about empathy in more depth in the conclusion. It is a myth that autistic people lack empathy.

> One reason why autistic people are seen as lacking emotional empathy is that autistic people don't generally express their empathy in the expected way, with body language, gesture, and statements such as "I'm sorry" or "I understand." An autistic person might express empathy by offering a solution to a problem, or by sharing a similar experience. Both of these can be seen as not validating the feelings of the other person.
>
> (Huston, 2021)

Autistic people will almost always refuse to engage in gossip. I am always the last person to know what is going on or what happened. We will not usually talk about people if they are not present. We find gossip morally grievous; we go directly to the person, or to a higher authority, about an issue if we have something to say. I remember a few years ago I tried to integrate and did the gossip thing with friends, and it seriously backfired; I am glad it did. It was wrong. I knew it was and I should not have done it. The last person you trust and gossip to is a gossiper!

At social events, especially foster carer support groups or foster carer coffee mornings, we all know gossip happens, be it about other foster carers, social workers, the local authority or fostering agency. When I would walk away or say I did not want to join in it did not help my integration into the group! It is another reason why autistic foster carers will not tend to thrive at a social event. If I need to say something or vent, I have my supervising social worker, or manager, or head of service, or Ofsted if needed. Autistic foster carers are not going to want to spend their time gossiping, moaning, or complaining to other foster carers. It is not interesting, or acceptable, or, frankly, helpful.

So, at any of these social activities I always appeared to be uncomfortable, stand-offish, awkward, and rude. I know this was not the outcome social services wanted for me when I attended one of their social engagements! I could not mingle and fit in properly. I would try to smile and nod, and need the toilet a lot, until I could leave.

I learned the best way to cope was to ask questions, lots of them, open-ended ones. I did not need to care about the answer, I would just nod and smile, and the person would be happy. People like to talk about themselves. So, I googled questions to ask people and memorised the best ones and once one had been answered I would throw in another quickly. After a while they would butterfly off to someone else and someone else would find me and I would repeat the whole routine.

If something unexpected happened – maybe someone got a chance to ask me a question or we had to get into groups and discuss something uninteresting, or we were told to do an icebreaker or a group team bonding activity – I was like a rabbit in the headlights. My nervous system would trigger, and I would go into flight or freeze mode. That made everyone uncomfortable, not just me!

I hated myself. Hated how I felt. Hated the hangover sensation, and my happiness and connection to those around me really were not being enhanced! I asked if I could stop going to these events but was told it was a "requirement", or there was a "non-discussional" expectation that we would be there.

As you can see, an occasion like Christmas dinner, or an event for foster carer appreciation, is an assault on all the senses, executive functioning, social and verbal communication. That is too overwhelming for many of us. It is a wonderful thing for social services to provide such events for most foster carers and I am thankful that they do. However, the thought is enough for me.

If social services can understand the above, then they are less likely to take offence if an autistic foster carer says, "No, I cannot come". As ever, not every autistic person is the same and some may enjoy the social aspect if it is an inclusive experience for them (McNulty, 2018).

Reasonable adjustments
Events and occasions

1. Offer the event or occasion but let your autistic foster carer know you do not expect them to come and that you are okay if they do not. Autistics feel sensitive to letting people down so to know they are not doing that will be great for the relationship.
2. Ask the autistic foster carer what you could put in place, if they would like to come, to make the time they spend there more enjoyable? A few changes could, maybe, make the event or occasion possible and enjoyable for some autistic foster carers.

A day trip out: too much – we will not have the spoons for it

1. We will not want our foster child or teenager to not participate in something they would love to do just because we cannot do it. If it is a day trip to Legoland or a big public

outing, perhaps someone else who is allowed to look after our child could go in our place. My mother used to take mine out on the big day trips. This concession worked well for everyone involved.

Training sessions

1. Is there a way to reduce sensory stimuli? Have a conversation with your autistic foster carers to see if there are any easy adjustments that could be made in the training room itself so it is more comfortable for them. They could visit the room with you beforehand and point out possible problems.
2. Is the icebreaker or team bonding exercise essential for the autistic foster carer to take part in? These are very stressful; we have come to focus and learn, and now social interaction and communication have also entered the arena. Can we be excused from that and go into another room or space for the ten minutes it will take?
3. If small group work is needed and the autistic foster carer is uncomfortable with social communication, can they become the note taker and be involved that way?
4. Changing seats or places can be a big disruption. If that is not an essential part of the training, is it possible to just stay in the seats we started in?
5. At lunch or in breaks are we able to take a timeout so we can rest rather than go through the small talk routine? Another option would be to have a "break-out", or "chill-out", room available.

    It is preferable that Break-Out Room/s and the Chill-Out Room are away from the Main Room – and with closeable doors – to prevent noise transfer.

Consider technology solutions that would enable participants to listen and/or watch the event via their own device. Alternatively, a feed (visual and sound) could be provided in a separate Break-Out Room. This would be beneficial for participants who may feel overwhelmed in the Main Room but do not want to be completely excluded.

A Chill-Out Room provides a quiet space for people to use if they need a break from the environment. Information about the location and use of the room should be provided in written material provided pre-event, as well as during the event introduction.

(Gatfield et al., 2018)

6. Knowing our senses can be hyper, someone in the training who starts clicking their biro or tapping their foot can become so loud on top of all the noise from the lights, electricity, general environment, PowerPoint clicker, aircon, etc., that we cannot concentrate. Leaders could say at the start that there is someone who is noise sensitive in the training, can we all be aware of the subconscious noises we make? This can really help eliminate those noises, enabling us to focus and learn without causing offence to anyone.

7. As an example of olfactory hypersensitivities, maybe a person with strong perfume will come and sit next to us in a meeting. If so, we will not be able to concentrate and we will need to move, which can be embarrassing. It is better to allow us to take our seats last because of this. I would always make sure I sat down after everyone else, pulling a chair to the back of the rows so I could sit by myself as this helped

my concentration. It can be easier for an autistic person to focus if they are not sitting next to someone.

Foster carer support groups

These monthly sessions really were impossible for me. Their function was to connect with people I did not know or need to know, and it was by small talk and gossip that this connection happened. An autistic foster carer is not likely to participate in "Have you heard?", or "What do you think about?" If we have an issue, we go to the top and do our best to sort it. We will not discuss it with someone who is unable to do anything.

Do these sessions have to be mandatory for an autistic foster carer? We all receive the minutes from the support groups. If there is something in the minutes that we either did not understand or had an opinion on we would be able to raise this with our supervising social worker. If your autistic foster carer asks to be excused from these meetings let them know that you want to understand why and anything they say is safe to share in a judgement-free space. If they let you know that small talk and the gossip side is too much, see if you can find alternative ways for them to receive the information, rather than take this the wrong way or make them attend the gatherings. Minutes worked perfectly for me.

Remembering that our main role is to be 100 per cent present to parent our child or teenager, simple changes can make all the difference. If allowances can be made for social events, and if reasonable adjustments can be made for training sessions, then social services are helping to equip us to be the best foster carers we can be.

5
Truth differences

I went into fostering alongside social services thinking I would fit in really well. Social services look after the most vulnerable children and their job is to ensure they are cared for in the best way possible. From the moment we start the fostering process there are key words that are said a lot: such as advocate, make a difference, and be child focused. Foster carers are told to tell the truth. It is one of the main points within the training to be a foster carer. We have to attend meetings, write reports, make weekly or monthly logs, and answer questions all the time. This is perfect for autistic people. We tend to be in pursuit of truth and totally understand the importance of these rules.

I can do everything that was asked of me so I felt that fostering would be a place where truth, honesty, and justice would thrive, and so would I. Surely this had to be the case because, working with our most vulnerable children, these are the very basic building blocks for their effective care.

I recently told a friend who fosters with a different local authority that I was writing this chapter and they replied, "Social services? Orwellian doublespeak is their language".

I was intrigued so I googled this. Wikipedia noted that: "The term 'doublespeak' derives from two concepts in George Orwell's novel *Nineteen Eighty-Four* ('Doublespeak', 2023)". Examples of doublespeak include use of euphemisms, jargon, vagueness, intentional omission, misdirection, and idioms in order to obscure the truth and engage in Machiavellian behaviour.

What shocked me was how I found these things to be very common in the way social services reacted to many issues over my years as a foster carer. This contradicted everything I had been told on the Journey into Fostering course, in fact what all foster carers are told, was the base line desire when fostering.

As we have seen in this book, the autistic pursuit of justice and truth is very strong. I am going to discuss some techniques which are normalised in my experiences with social services professionals. I will give examples of these techniques happening to me so that it is not just theory which we can ignore. Unfortunately, they all too often easily slipped into common practice. I will explain how these techniques affect the autistic foster carer and finally give some simple ways to make reasonable adjustments.

In writing this chapter I have been flooded with emotion. Even today I am asking, "Why?" Not a logical "why?" I understand why they did it. But why would one adult be okay with using a tactic which they knew would hurt another adult?

The singer, Pink, recently released a song called "Hate Me" and the lyrics are pertinent to this chapter for me. I have had it on repeat and this song has been therapy while writing this chapter, trying to make the nonsensical make sense. This is the reality of an autistic foster carer facing these tactics. Maybe, before you read any further, listen to that song and have it in your mind as you read the following examples.

> Truth differences 61

Gaslighting

This is when you are made to question yourself. The National Bullying Helpline website says:

> Psychologists describe gaslighting as a subtle but unhealthy manipulative behaviour. An employee who is the subject of gaslighting will likely, certainly initially, struggle to understand what is occurring – similar to Bergman's character in the film.
> Typically, an employee cannot "put their finger on the problem" …
> Gaslighting is classic abuse of power. It is bullying. It's a manipulate [sic] power-game, which individuals or groups of individuals play within a workplace with deliberate intent to control an individual or control a situation. A perpetrator could be a co-worker or a line manager. However, gaslighting may be cultural, i.e., from the top down, condoned at Corporate Management level. It is an entirely unacceptable, subtle, management style.
>
> (National Bullying Helpline, 2022)

After I had an allegation (see Chapter 6), had been through autistic burnout, and had come out the other side, an agency fostering authority of mine said they wanted me to see a linked professional to work through my feelings. I did not see why I needed to. The situation had been completed for over three months by this time. It was over. It was sorted. I had moved on. I had no feelings except for being bored with my agency for still talking about it and telling me how hard it must have been for me. Yes, it had been hard, but it was finished. I could not hold on to it. It was not safe for me to hold on to it. I looked back to an email I wrote to the linked professional in which I tried to explain that I had no emotional residue. I was simply bored with it all. I wrote:

> I know if I say I don't need therapy then that can get decided that it's proof that I do. Lol! So I appreciate I am caught here! I know I don't have a choice to attend but it's a full-on waste of your, the agency and my time and resources as I'm so over this and moved on… bored is my feeling and I'm way more resilient than folk think!!! I am super open with my feelings and told everyone my feeling journey as I had them over this past 9 months. Everyone knows my feelings and how they changed and what I felt pretty much followed the grief pattern in hindsight. I felt them, worked through them and my only feeling now is boredom when talking about it. I'm genuinely so bored of it I have no other feelings. I can't sustain 9 months of energy on something that pointless if I'm honest, I've got bigger and awesome things to do with my time and energy with work and charity, so it would be negative and victim mentality to sit and mope about something as stupid as this has been. And I don't really have that in me. I'm a move on, not a "dwell on pointless" person. I decided basically my choice was, A- it was a mess up, can't be undone, move on and get over it. Or B- leave Fostering if it annoyed me that much. I still have feelings for Fostering so choose to move on and get over it. If anything, Fostering lost a good carer for 9 months, that's their loss not mine. Hope that helps understand where I am coming from. Oh, and if it's because I didn't tell them in the meeting

> what my feelings were when asked, that was because I was not going to let them use unethical yet obvious techniques before an interrogation. They aren't silly. They know if they get someone to invest in feelings before the questioning that person is unsettled. I found it funny that they even tried it to be honest. But I wasn't going to play the game, I had a list of points to get across and that was one of them… It wasn't for any other reason that I refused.
>
> (Tanner, personal communication)

Wordy it may have been, but I felt I had clearly explained that I had moved on. I expected them to do the same!

The linked professional wrote back, explaining that after reading my email they still felt it would be beneficial to have a couple of sessions to explore what I had shared. I replied:

> You wrote that you felt it would be beneficial to explore what I shared in my email. In my eyes I was trying to explain to neurotypicals that I'm bored. I explained it in numerous ways in the hope one way made sense. Please let me know what needs exploring as I think I'm totally open re: feelings. I know for a fact until now folk have probably wished I keep my feelings and truths to myself LOL, so why are my feelings not being believed now? I feel that if my email isn't taken on face value and something in it makes folk feel I have an issue, then we have a communication problem and misrepresentation. I'm 10000% truthful and honest. I'm bored and healthily worked through my feelings and moved on. If [my agency] don't believe my first email re: being bored and having worked through it all

then I don't really want to justify or prove myself. I'm not into proving myself... I'm into expressing my truth and having a trust relationship both ways. I can't play a game or do something that is annoying. And this is annoying. [my agency] need to move on, like I have. This is an agency problem not mine and I don't like the transference. Sorry but that's my final decision.

(Tanner, personal communication)

Thankfully, the agency authority then replied and said it was okay, I did not need to go to therapy!

I really could not understand what was happening. Why were the agency authority and their linked professional trying to make it look as if I was still emotionally affected by the situation? It had ended three months previously and many ebbs and flows of life's tides had happened in those three months. It was in the past. I had been clear that I had worked through my feelings at the time, during those nine months of the protracted allegation. My only feeling genuinely was being bored of still talking about it even though it was over. I had made it clear that I saw that a tactic was being played in this meeting, but I could not put my finger on it. I just knew I had no intention of speaking about my past feelings at that time. I had important points to make, which they were aware of. I needed to stay focused, not be taken off track by speaking about historic emotions.

I spoke to a friend about how confused I felt over this. They explained that this was normal. They had clearly messed up so much with the allegation situation that they had to look as if they were doing something positive for me in the aftermath. The friend continued that they needed me to be emotionally traumatised so they could offer therapy and "look good and caring". This whole episode was about them covering their backs and controlling a situation, so they came out smelling of roses. My friend also told me I had "outed" a technique they used in meetings to dysregulate people. They probably wanted to "reframe" my opinion on both the technique, and the reason why they did it, to something more palatable for them as it was not a good look when it was stated as fact, as I had done.

Gaslighting is controlling an individual or a situation to the point that the individual knows something is wrong but cannot put their finger on it. I was not emotionally traumatised at that point. They were trying to make me believe I was. A very common technique used!

Twisting

At one time in particular, I had a manager within social services who I found very difficult to cope with. She used most of the tactics in this chapter and she would only ever communicate over the phone, so that I had no evidence of anything she was saying to me. If I told anybody else in social services about the conversations, she would deny everything. So, after one phone call where I was given a threat of having a child moved to a residential unit, I lost my cool. I apologised and asked that in future all communication with her should be written so that we would not be in that position again. I had asked for what I believed to be a reasonable adjustment. I could not cope with the phone calls and no evidence of what was being said with this manager. I believed email communication would resolve this and suggested this as a way to move forward. This was then twisted.

It was written in a report that I had described how I responded to "social care professionals" following the discussion about the possibility of moving my then foster child to a residential unit. I had, apparently, acknowledged that I did not react well in my response, due to the strong emotions this suggestion had evoked for me. I was purported to have said that I felt this created tension in my working relationship with "social care" and afterwards, it continued, "she said she did not wish to have any further phone communication, because she was keen to have a written record of any communication going forward".

My response was very clear. While I agreed with the essence of the final statement I explained: "I believe I did not say Social Care – I said [manager's first name]". I went on to explain that I was perfectly happy to communicate by phone with all of the social workers and I did not have any tension in my working relationships with anyone other than [manager's first name]. It was [manager's first name] that I wanted to have email communication with following previous meetings which caused me serious problems. I even asked them to check with the IRO (independent reviewing officer) if necessary as she was aware of this situation. I continued that it was not fair to make it sound as if I had said it was all of social services as I had not. I reiterated that I needed emails in this specific case only, to ensure all conversations had a written record so that I felt that there was accountability for both of us. I understood their desire to keep this non-personal, but on that point it did not work.

My words had been twisted to make something sound very different from what it was. My words were exaggerated to "professionals" and "Social Care" when I had asked for this to apply to just one person. This was then written down in my permanent record giving a very different take on what had happened. It protected the manager in question and made me, as the foster carer, sound binary and excessive, suggesting that I had issue with everyone in social services. Therefore, the problem was the foster carer's, that is, mine, and social services did not need to look into any unprofessionalism on the part of their manager.

Triangulation

This is when, if two people disagree, say a social service manager and a foster carer, the manager will bring in a third party and this third party will either show agreement with the manager or deliver the manager's message. This third party will be someone the foster carer likes or trusts so the foster carer will question less. Social workers would often do this with my teenagers if they knew the teenager was not going to accept the information they wanted to give. I would be brought in to back up the social worker. Sometimes this is well intentioned and helpful but, on other occasions, it is not used for positive reasons.

Intentional omissions

Something that is intentional is deliberate, decided, chosen. Omission is something left out, as in not included or not done. Social services fostering social workers do this both verbally and in writing when it suits their purpose. As we can see with many of the examples in this chapter alone, intentional omission pops up quite regularly. If something crops up that does not suit the agenda or the objective you will not find it in any subsequent report.

Projection

This is when a person puts their personal feelings or characteristics onto someone else. In the minutes from one meeting a manager noted that the social worker I was interacting with was very clear but also quite direct in her approach while I, apparently, was not! It was suggested that these different characteristics may have resulted in occasions where the social worker and I "misconstrued each other".

My response:

> Once again, if this was said [in the meeting], I would have challenged this – especially, "Social worker is very clear but also quite direct in her approach and Megan does not present like this". What does this mean? That I do not present in a direct way? I have numerous emails clearly stating exactly what I am thinking / needing / asking, etc., all of which were and are available for anyone to see. I am very direct and this comment needs to be explained as I would like to know what it means.
>
> (Tanner, personal communication)

This really is the height of gaslighting and projection. Telling an autistic person that they do not present as clearly and directly in their approach as a neurotypical social worker does is, frankly, laughable. And that is the reason behind statements being misconstrued does not hold water. First, had this statement been made in the meeting, which I assure you it was not, everyone there would have questioned it as, if anything, I am generally too open and direct and this is what can cause issues. For this statement to be written in the minutes of a meeting when, categorically, it was never said during that meeting, is concerning.

Out of interest, you might notice I start my response with, "Once again, if this was said". This strongly suggests that there were previous comments in the minutes about things which had not been said in the meeting. Minutes should be just that. Factual representations of each part of the discussion. There should be no additions, and there would, under normal conditions, be the option to disagree with them and have that noted. There was no such option here. I honestly have no words sometimes!

Name calling

This is when a person uses some characteristic about another person in a negative way. I am looking at a document now where a social worker or manager has written "she is too dramatic" when talking about me. I think by dramatic they mean blunt and truthful, in which case they are correct because the truth, sadly, can be dramatic when it is said out loud and not twisted for an ulterior motive. But name calling is used to make a person feel of lower status, or that they have problems, or that the person is not on the same level of intellect, ability, or professionalism as the speaker.

As a foster carer I would never have been allowed to call an individual social worker dramatic, or emotional, or awkward, even if I thought it. But they were able to use such terms regularly about foster carers. "He is a bit awkward", or "She is good but very emotional". On this point I noticed that social services were far more willing to use this about their female foster carers than their male foster carers. There is an interesting point to ponder!

Female foster carers were often spoken of as dramatic, emotional, difficult, tiresome, to name a few epithets I heard professionals use openly. There was, apparently, no problem with this. It was normalised and accepted behaviour. It was not alright, however, for it to be done the other way round, by foster carers with regard to social workers, which is also something to ponder!

Theories treated as fact

I had a comment written about me suggesting that I would not want to adopt, as a single foster carer, in case I met someone. This was said about me in a meeting that I was not invited to. I was not asked personally about it. However, it was discussed by a group of professionals, they came up with this idea between themselves, decided it was a rather good hypothesis and, therefore, it became a "fact" without me ever even knowing it had been said until years later. This is an example of an outrageous discussion and decision being made without any input from the foster carer involved. Theory treated as fact.

On another occasion, when discussing my thoughts on a particular foster child who was showing signs of severe trauma, it was decided that I was becoming fearful at home as I did not know what (XX) was capable of doing. I apparently stated that I had been naïve about (XX's) past during some meeting I had had with a particular social worker.

When I read this, I responded: "I am not fearful – that is an unfair exaggeration. I never stated I was naive about XX's past – this is untrue, and the implications of this sentence are unfair". Again, this was a theory someone had evoked without checking it with me and it became a written fact in a permanent report even though it had never been stated by me.

Thankfully, sometimes, other professionals step in on behalf of the foster carer during meetings. These three sentences were said about me when I was not present to answer them. All were theories, or personal feelings and thoughts stated as facts. I had never been questioned on these points to see if they were true and only found out about them sometime later. This time there was a linked professional at the meeting who could refute the arguments on my behalf and, thankfully, did. The statements about my relationship with my foster child stated:

- She doesn't know any of XX friends.
- She talks too late at night with XX, why isn't she putting her to bed?
- She thinks she's a therapist.

The linked professional replied:

1. "'She doesn't know any of XX friends"

The linked professional explained that I had always been aware of a great number of XX's friends in their sessions with me; aware of their characteristics, the ever-changing relationships between them and XX; their arguments and good times. They continued: "This statement is false".

2. "She talks too late at night with XX, why isn't she putting her to bed?"

The linked professional recalled the incident which was being spoken about when I and XX had talked for half an hour after XX had come down saying they could not sleep and were thinking about traumatic things. They explained that I had shared this with this professional to ensure they had a better picture of how XX was dealing with their trauma.

3. "She thinks she's a therapist."

The linked professional then explained that, far from being in the wrong, I parented therapeutically, which was what all foster carers and adopters were encouraged to do, although many are unable to. They then told the meeting that their professional role was created to help carers and adopters do this, as therapeutic parenting 24/7 could help shift things substantially compared to therapy once a week, especially due to the importance of the carer/parent–child relationship.

I can never thank this linked professional enough.

Labelling

In social services children and foster carers are labelled all too often. It is normalised and the consequences and harm it does are never considered. Throughout this book we can see how many times I was labelled. Labelling is an extension of name calling. It starts by adding adjectives to a foster carer's name, creating characteristics that then become their label. It is also very dehumanising.

Changing minds, or information, without telling anyone – making the new information the only information

When we begin the fostering journey we complete a Form F. This holds all the information about you. But the question is, does anyone actually read it? Some years into my fostering career I called out a bad practice issue, and suddenly, things began to be said about me which had no link to reality. In one report at this time, written by a child social worker, queries were raised about my name change. I had said, according to them, that I had been bullied at school and was returning to [live in] W.., and as I was an actress I wanted to change my name. However, they continued, it was not able to be followed up due to conflicting accounts from both myself and my assessing social worker.

I amended this document as it bore no resemblance to the truth.

> Who did I say this to? I was never bullied at school, in fact quite the opposite. Please see from my FORM F the Assessing Social Worker X's comments on attachment B. No. I changed my surname in 1998 after my parents divorced as is correctly accounted for in my FORM F, and I changed my first name when I became an actress in 2001 for Equity. I moved to W….. in 2011, 10 whole years after I changed my name."
>
> (Tanner, personal communication)

As you can see in the reply, there was no conflict between the assessing social worker and myself. But, although my Form F had been done so many years previously, and I had had multiple children and child social workers since, this child social worker felt she could say this. She had clearly never read my Form F; she had no idea who the assessor was or what had been written. Possibly she jumped to wrong conclusions because she had not checked the facts.

This "concern" suddenly popped up, but it had never been a concern or issue before this child social worker needed to create one. The easy and honest answer to why I had changed my name was in the Form F in total agreement with my assessing social worker. The child social worker wrote their own words and, by doing so, made me sound historically unreliable, untruthful, and giving "conflicting" information. In a short meeting, none of the professionals are going to do background checks to make sure that this child social worker was being honest. Therefore, they could and did discredit what I was trying to point out as a problem in the system at that time. They had no actual evidence or reason or ability to make me look that way, so they changed the information and this became the new reality.

After the meeting I wrote a ten-page document with verifiable amendments to everything this child social worker had written. I was then told my amendments would not be entered into the file. Her document was entered. Mine, with all the corrections, was not because the meeting had been held and completed.

Being autistic and having a strong sense of justice this caused me serious upset and confusion. As with all of these tactics, they mentally damage autistic people because we just are not able to do them ourselves and we cannot make them make sense. I know for many days and weeks after this meeting I was like a hamster on a wheel asking my support group over and over again, "Why did they say this? Why did they do this?" It took weeks for my support group to bring me down.

Using threats or coercion

Many times, if my child or teenager was displaying behaviours that social services did not like, they, and I, would be threatened with them being removed and put into a residential unit. I would say most of my children and teenagers were threatened with this possibility to their face by their child social workers at some time or another. I found it horrifying that a child as young as 8, or a teen as old as 17, would be told this option, but it was normalised behaviour. However, it was not considered to be threatening, merely fact. It was considered to be acceptable. This was actually raised by a linked professional who wrote in their report, "We made both [child's name] and Megan feel unsafe, with 'threats' that if the child runs away again, we shall have to consider residential care". This linked professional even wrote the word "threat".

Threatening will never help a child or a foster carer. It increases stress levels and for an autistic foster carer this is very harmful.

Disregarding verifiable facts

Many times I was accused of things I did, or did not do, and I could prove the accusation wrong. My responses and evidence were hardly ever added into reports.

I was taken ill. In an email it was stated that I had failed on at least one occasion to let the local authority know about things that had occurred. The example given was that I had failed to let my supervising social worker know that I had suspected appendicitis.

My supervising social worker was also off sick that day. Despite a hospital trip, I had phone records of me messaging the on-call social worker to explain what had happened. They were dated and timed. I also had a text message from them acknowledging my message! In it they clearly said they were sorry to hear about my appendix problem, wished me well, and asked me to keep them updated. They even told me not to worry as they would sort it out when I felt better. It ended, "Take care". How had I failed to let them know? Was this evidence taken into account to rectify the error? Sadly, no.

Another example was written in an email by a social worker, sent out in November, although I cannot remember why. It stated that I provided discrepant points of view to different individuals at social services or that I kept changing my story. The only example provided by the social worker was that I had given an incorrect date in a conversation at one time. I responded:

> Please see below the email where I clearly correct the date mistake. Social Worker came for supervision on 16th Sep. and I gave an incorrect date and I emailed on 18th Sep. when I realised my mistake. Please see highlighted paragraph.
> 18/09
> Hello – little email to hopefully settle any worries or concerns.
> Ohhh. Firstly I need to change some info I gave you on Tues as I was wrong!! When you spoke about the concern over xx running through the kitchen window before I woke up, I said xx must have done this ages ago, prob in May. I got this wrong – they went through the window morning of Friday 1 Aug.
>
> (Tanner, personal communication)

My email explaining my mistake had been sent just two days after the initial conversation, as soon as I realised what I had done. The complaint about the incorrect date was written two months after it had been rectified.

I was told that my rectification was disregarded. My reminder that I had rectified it and the proof would not enter into any amendment of the written record. By not entering my amendments, verifiable facts were ignored, in this case making me seem to use incorrect information. Not only is this wrong, but, for an autistic foster carer, this is so damaging.

Misdirection

Dictionary.com says misdirection is "the use of misleading appearances or distraction to prevent detection of one's true intent" (Dictionary.com, 2023). We get false statements being written about foster carers and children regularly and never corrected. This chapter is littered with a few examples of mine! Although I was able to show proof, none of my replies made any difference. These statements are still there about me as if I have never challenged anything. This misleading information was used to distract either from what I was trying to bring to light at the time or prevent detection of a professional's true intent. Misdirection.

When I transferred from my local authority to an agency the agency needed to see my file and had emailed many times asking for it. They were not able to continue my transfer until they had seen it. So, tired of this impasse, I eventually wrote again to the manager of my local authority, adding in the head of service:

> I have just spoken to X at [the agency] and they have said they need to see my file from the LA and that that hasn't been possible to achieve as yet. My application to foster with them cannot go any further until they have seen my file and it has now been a few months since [the agency] made a first request to the LA to see it. I need this swiftly sorted. They are aware that the LA and I have had differences and that my file may well be quite questionable, so if this is the reality, and the delay is due to this, please do not worry, they are aware of my concern around this, so it is not a problem.
>
> (Tanner, personal communication)

I received a reply from the manager telling me that they did not know that I had applied to (agency name) to become a foster carer. To their knowledge no one from (agency name) has spoken to them about seeing my file. They went on to say that if the agency would like to contact them – preferably by email – they would arrange a time for someone to come to the office to see my file.

Of course, the manager knew. I had made sure, unequivocally, that this communication had, in fact, taken place. I had emailed and told her. They also knew me only too well. This misdirection was obvious. They were suggesting that the agency was lying. That they had not actually asked for the file over the months they told me they had been asking for it. But why use misdirection? With our rocky past surely they should have been pleased that I was going to move to an agency.

As we are learning in this book there are consequences for standing up to power. And that was something I did whenever it was needed. Making things take longer than needed, holding up processes and timeframes and causing frustration are petty ways to give a consequence. The requests had clearly been received but ignored, and that was to be the status quo for as long as possible. By now I understood this, which was why I had added the head of service into the email. I knew I would be ignored by the manager; the agency would be ignored; but hoped that if the head of service knew what was going on action would finally happen.

And guess what? The Agency received my file in response to this final email interaction. I went on to foster many other children from the local authority over the years.

How this looks in practice as an autistic foster carer in social services

We are mandated to advocate and speak "truth". This means that sometimes we have to make a stand and have different views from social workers.

> If you take a stand against management as an individual, you are likely to feel the full repercussions for doing so.
> (Foster Care Workers Union, n.d.)

> Reporting a concern to your provider or raising an issue that could have or is having a detrimental effect on you as a foster carer, your foster child or a young person, can be a tricky and daunting process.
> (FosterWiki, 2021)

> Foster carers are long overdue their own voice.
>
> (FosterWiki, 2021)

> Foster carers regularly find information written and recorded about them that is not correct or is false.
>
> (FosterWiki, 2021)

> We see the same issues and concerns arising and we see the constant struggle that foster carers encounter to have their voices heard and their knowledge and professional skills respected.
>
> (Foster Support, 2022)

All of these quotes are saying that, sadly, within the system, the truth is not required. If we tell the truth as a foster carer, there will be a backlash. We were told at the beginning of our journey into fostering that truthfulness is imperative in fostering, yet we quickly learn that this is not so. We must lie or we will face consequences. Also lies will be told about us and we must accept that.

False statements are written about foster carers and never corrected. Although I was able to show proof, or to reply to comments, most of my replies did not make any difference. These statements are still there about me in various documents as if I have never disproved or challenged anything.

The impact these things have on an autistic foster carer is incredibly painful. The vagueness, intentional omission, misdirection, gaslighting, projection, and so on, in order to obscure the truth, fits well with Orwellian doublespeak. It causes mental health issues, sleep issues, anxiety, PTSD, and depression for the foster carers.

Now for autistic foster carers, who we have already learned tend to have a very high faith and belief in truth and justice, this is nearly impossible to get their heads around.

When we look at impulse inhibition, meltdown, or shutdown, everything in this chapter is going to spark that in an autistic foster carer. We cannot cope with this style of behaviour. When we challenge, or refute, or prove it to be false, it does not go in our favour. It is turned against us.

An autistic foster carer has to mask continuously, but in the face of these behaviours, the mask is not going to happen.

Autistic foster carers are unlikely to quit because we have a tenacious perseverance and a belief that things will get better. Just over a year into fostering, I learned that everyone else who started fostering at the same time as I had quit. After a year or less I was the only one left. They gave up because they could not cope with the system. Autistic foster carers will tend to stay and they will experience mental health problems if social services continue to use these unethical, unprofessional behaviours.

> From what I've heard in large circles, by and large, autistics don't want to leave their place of employment but **feel forced to leave**. Often coping with debilitating anxiety and PTSD, autistic community members state that it is the repeated incidents of bullying, segregation, misunderstandings, discrimination, and other oppressive workplace practices that they find intolerable.

> It's not pretty, but it needs to be said. This is the world we live in. It's not the autism; it's the workplace culture.
>
> (Ciampi, 2019)

> While all workers suffer the negative effects of bullying, these effects are often particularly detrimental to autistic individuals. Autistic people are more likely to have chronic autonomic nervous system (ANS) hyperarousal – a chronic biological threat response. This makes autistic individuals more vulnerable to harmful physiological stress response to bullying and incivility, possibly resulting in physical illness or even cardiac events.
>
> (Praslova, 2022)

We can see in this chapter how an autistic foster carer can be dehumanised. Being dehumanised, misrepresented, or vilified may cover professionals' backs; it may distract from the issues that the autistic foster carer has pointed out rather than having those issues dealt with; but through this the autistic foster carer is destroyed and the damage done is immense. These tactics, although normalised, are cruel and have long-lasting impact, long after the social worker or manager even remembers the report they wrote or the words they said.

Social services is fully aware of all forms of abuse. It is there to protect children from abuse. That is what it is intended to do. However, there is also a need to protect autistic foster carers from psychological abuse from social services staff. Wikipedia notes that "*Psychological abuse*, often called *emotional abuse* …, may include bullying, gaslighting, and abuse in the workplace".

If the examples I have used were the only ones encountered in over a decade I could think, "Fair play". But they were not. If you need to use these tactics, trust me, there is something going on that is rotten, because, if there was not, you would not need to use them. Please listen to the lyrics of the Pink song, "Hate Me". These lyrics will be the residue that is left on the autistic foster carer. We need to have true compassion for this in order to make lasting changes in these attitudes.

Reasonable adjustments

I do not think I can even write this section! It is simple. Do not do these things. Do not do it to anyone. Know that if you use these insidious, normalised, abhorrent behaviours, you are causing harm mentally and emotionally to an autistic foster carer and no professional has the right to do that to another person.

1. If we are in a "curated" truth meeting, rather than a "truth" meeting, we will need breaks to process information, so we do not become emotional. If we ask for a break let us take it. We become emotional when things are not in alignment.
2. *Do not use psychologically abusive tactics.* Autistics generally have no ability to use or understand them.

6
Rule differences

Autistic foster carers will generally follow rules to the letter. By nature, we tend to be rule followers. Rules help us navigate our pathway through the veritable minefield of living in a neurotypical world and ensure we do the "right thing". On the flip side of this, however, those rules have to make sense. If they do not, or are arbitrary, we will ignore them as being irrelevant. So being a rule follower and a rule breaker for us are both equally true as seen in these quotes.

> Rules can be very important for some Autistic people. It may be difficult for an autistic person to take a different approach to something once they have been taught the "right" way to do it.
>
> (National Autistic Society, 2020a)

Autistic people tend to respond well to set ways of working and routines. This would appear to be a bonus in the workplace – and it can be, but the rules have to make sense.

> When an autistic person develops a routine that they strictly adhere to, it makes sense to them at some level. When they have to fit into a routine that someone else has developed, and the rules seem arbitrary, it can be especially hard for an autistic person to accept, likely

due to the cognitive inflexibility that is a characteristic of autism.

(Jack, 2022)

When it came to safeguarding children in my care, even if I felt the rule was ridiculous, I would not break it. Safeguarding is safeguarding; you cannot blur the lines. Or can you?

Is it or is it not a rule?

In our "Journey to Foster" training back in 2011, when I was starting the process to become a foster carer, we were told that if a child was sick you could not sit on their bed. If you read a bedtime story to a child, you must sit on a chair a few feet away from the bed. The bed was off limits at all times – for safeguarding purposes you may never sit on it.

I questioned this. If the child was young and needed comfort how was this holistic parenting? It did not matter. The rule was the rule and I was just starting out so I was determined to follow it to the letter, even though I disagreed.

A few months later I had my first young foster child and, as luck would have it, they got sick. I called a social worker saying I felt very unkind letting the child be sick and not sitting next to them, stroking their hair or giving them comfort. The chair a few feet away was not a good place to show love to a sick child. The social worker replied, "Oh, sit on the bed. Everyone does it".

This blew my brain! The rule had been told to us as being a firm, safeguarding rule, a protection against abuse of the child. It had been relayed to us in a non-negotiable tone. Now I was hearing that, in practice, no one listens to the rule, it was not important and I could break it.

It went further. I was then told as the conversation progressed, "Yes, everyone does it, but I suggest you don't mention it or write it in your log, of course".

So, during one conversation, I was told first to break the rule, sit on the bed and give comfort, and, secondly, told not to write it up in my logs, but to keep it quiet! I was to break two rules in one go – (1) the bed rule and (2) the open honesty rule. I was informed I could lie in my logs, or at the very least, use intentional omission.

So, now the question was, "Just how important is the don't lie rule? I am allowed to lie sometimes but not at other times. But how do I know when to choose?" For me, as an autistic foster carer, this was completely confusing and concerning.

(This was back in 2012. I believe this "bed rule" has changed over the years since then. But there will be many other examples of "is it a rule or not?" that will validate my point today, I am sure.)

Policy and procedure rules

As in any system there are specific procedures and policies for things that may happen. Let's take allegations as an example because, in my mind, allegations are of serious importance, both for child safeguarding and for foster carer mental health.

Most foster carers, if they foster a child who can talk, will face allegations. As an aside I had a child abscond and called the police following the rules. This policeman also knew I was the founder of a charity which works in Africa with the mission to end child abuse. At the end of the phone call the policeman said, "I'm a foster carer too. Can I give you some advice? Only foster children who can't walk and can't talk. This is for your safety as allegations are going to happen otherwise. My wife and I only foster babies". Years later I still think about his advice! How true it was.

So, a few years ago I had a historical allegation made against me. This means an allegation was made about something which had allegedly happened some years previously. This is important to note. Allegations can be backdated. Children are going to make allegations, some will be true, but some will be because the child wants something or is angry with a situation. This allegation was easily proven to not be possible. I even sent video evidence. So I was not worried at all. I believed it would be sorted out in a few weeks with no problem as there was copious evidence to show it could not have happened.

However, I soon became aware that policy and procedure rules are equally as elastic as the tell the truth rule. We should look at the policy surrounding an allegation. My local authority website has its policy and procedure advice online. (I have not added the link to safeguard my local authority.) Following an allegation, the policy is: a strategy meeting should be held "within 2 working days".

According to the report from my fostering agency the allegation was made on 5 August. Following policies and procedures I should have expected a strategy meeting within two working days, so by 7 August. However, on 8 September an email was sent by my agency to the local authority suggesting a strategy meeting be held as this had not yet happened.

Two days? That is over a month and, note, this was an email suggesting that this should be done, not an actual meeting.

On 13 November there was a strategy meeting, however, my fostering agency report states, "This was to conclude the section 47 investigation. The initial meeting had taken place on 10/11/2020 but [agency name] had not been invited to this". In the local authority strategy meeting policy point 3.2 says, "the following people will be invited. f. Any other agency involved with the child or foster family".

My agency should have been invited and were not. This was now 14 weeks from the allegation and 9 weeks from the email suggesting a strategy meeting, clearly not within two working days as the policy states.

On 16 November, a few days after this strategy meeting, my agency asked for the minutes. They repeated this request on 26 November and, finally, on 14 December they made the local authority aware that the investigation would be completed the following day, without having had sight of those minutes. By the time the final report was written and signed no one had seen the minutes of this strategy meeting. It had taken place without all of the parties involved taking part, 14 weeks after the allegation was first raised.

I eventually received the report on 20 December, again over a month since the last documented interaction that was listed in the report.

So that would be the end of it, you might imagine, but you would be wrong. After all, everyone agreed the allegation was unsubstantiated. But I was then told there had to be a meeting with me before I could be put back on the referral list and this could not happen until 2 March, over two months away.

I still could not foster until that meeting had been held, even though the decision that the allegation was totally unsubstantiated had been made. Where is that timeline in the policy and procedures? It is not!

But this is what happens when you upset people in social services, and I did upset people. Because the timings did not follow the rules I complained. I even got my local Member of Parliament involved to try to get accountability so that the policy was followed. It is openly acknowledged by a huge percentage of foster carers and foster carer support systems that if you stand up to make a positive change you will face consequences. Mine was an extra two months of delay before being able to foster again!

As a foster carer who dealt with highly traumatised children and teenagers, I was put on hold for 30 weeks for something that I could absolutely prove never happened, could not physically have happened, in fact, something which was literally impossible, and which most of those involved in the subsequent investigations agreed from the start could not have happened.

As soon as this final meeting took place referrals came in. I went on to foster three more teenagers over the next few years, but that 30 weeks of my life was, with no exaggeration, a living hell. Everyone told me to leave fostering. The damage it did to my mental health while I tried to get my head around how no policy and procedure was being followed was intense (see Chapter 7).

I wrote to many people during those weeks and months asking for help, including my local Member of Parliament. He did contact my local authority and got a response on 24 November stating that many social workers and managers involved in the situation had left during this time, which was why it was taking so long. When we looked more deeply into this it became clear that this was not actually the full reason, but it worked as a misdirection at the time. Furthermore, my autistic brain asked,

> If a social worker or manager is going to start a historical allegation and then leave how the heck can all T's not be crossed and I's not be dotted for their successor on the off chance that this historical allegation is founded? Where is the safeguarding for the child in this? How can this excuse be used as a reason? Why was this excuse not a red flag?
>
> (Tanner, personal communication)

When I asked my agency who had made the final decision, they told me it was the local authority. When I asked the local authority about it, they told me it was my agency. I went back to the agency, and they gave me a very unclear retraction of their previous statement. It was very woolly and incoherent. In fact, the whole thing was the biggest "pig's ear"! Luckily, in this case, it was not a proven allegation, but what security could I find in the policy and procedures that are there to safeguard children and foster carers following this?

Both the local authority and my fostering agency were party to these failings.

> Research has shown 78% of allegations are unsubstantiated or unfounded, yet leave devastation in their wake, their impact should never be

underestimated as carers are left with no voice, scared, powerless, shamed and judged.

(FosterWiki, 2023)

This finding reiterated the messages from the State of the Nation's Foster Care 2021 thematic report on allegations (The Fostering Network, 2021).

General rules on children or teenagers

Rules are not only given to foster carers by social services. There are many rules put on our foster children and teenagers which do not make sense.

At one point I had a 17-year-old who was told by their child social worker that they had a 9 p.m. curfew. They constantly broke the curfew, and I was told that, every time they did, I had to call the police. It was crazy. I asked if we could stop the curfew because "force equals resistance". We were asking for this teenager to rebel. Their friends would not be out much, if any, later, so did we need to enforce it? I was told that I needed to show strength, and the teenager needed to learn that "they didn't make the rules".

Now, I will be honest. I had learned ten years previously from the "sitting on the bed" rule that some rules are to be broken and you may deliberately omit any knowledge of that happening. So, I applied that rule here. I went ahead and cancelled the curfew, after which my teenager was always back home by 9.30 p.m. at the latest. I asked them why, when they could stay out all night? Their answer? "I was bored." The only reason they broke the curfew was rebellion; take it away and they had nothing to rebel against and the problem was solved.

I can decide to break a rule, but I cannot do the intentional omission part. That is going too far for my autistic brain. So I logged what I had done and told the social worker that I had defied them. Even though the problem was solved, and I was not needing to call the police every night, I was told that it was disappointing that I had not followed the guidance – the guidance which was unhelpful and causing problems. Social services wanted the foster carer, in this instance me, to be obedient rather than problem solving.

We see this many times when we look into the rules we are told to use with our children or teenagers. Social workers think they know best because of the training they have, but they do not live with the individual child or teenager and do not have to live with the consequences of arbitrary rules. I feel sure the police were relieved when the nightly calls stopped as well.

Timeframe rules

In the chapter on executive functioning we saw that a "two hour" supervision time might be better if it simply finishes when it has fulfilled what it set out to do, be that 45 minutes, or less, or more. So, do these timeframe rules need to be fixed or can they be flexible for autistic foster carers? I would suggest flexibility would lead to more depth in the discussions and a better relationship between the carer and their social worker.

Communication rule

One unspoken rule is the communication rule. Without it being said, it is apparent that we must all communicate in the neurotypical way. This was written in one of my reports as a negative by a social worker about me, "Her emails are too dramatic, things are awful and then they're OK again".

I fully agree with them! I would not use the word dramatic as that was intentionally meant to be a put down. But, yes, when things are awful, for example my child is investing in risky behaviours and I am finding that I am not able to help them make more positive choices, I will certainly send emails asking for advice, support, help for the child or me so we can protect the child from themselves. If I am being ignored, or getting nowhere, the information in the email will be "dramatic" because the danger level of the risky behaviour is "dramatic". There is an urgency to help this child and, unfortunately, three weeks waiting time for any reply is not acceptable.

However, once I have finally been listened to and we have made headway, guess what, all is OK again, because my child is OK and not doing things that could result in tragic endings! And I am not able to hold on to something after it is finished.

When I am trying to get a nine-month allegation situation or an unfair personal representation sorted you bet my communication will be black and white and not carefully couched as expected by social services.

Dramatic? I do not think that would be the correct term. More likely blunt, honest, and truthful. But, once everything is sorted out, yes, I will be OK again because things have been resolved and made right. That is the important thing here, made right. If social services creates rules and procedures then they should adhere to them.

Social services is a "status-driven" organisation. Foster carers are generally called "the foster carer", not by name. To be fair this is slowly changing. Professionals means social workers, psychologists, in fact, anyone working in the system but the foster carers. We are not classed as professionals or treated as equals.

> These changes include foster carers needing to manage increasing levels of complex behaviour and presentations, to work more inclusively and closely with birth families and social workers, and to participate in more formal tasks such as care planning, record keeping and attending meetings, as well as being subjected to greater monitoring and regulation. It has been argued that this has resulted in a trend towards "professionalisation" in foster care.
>
> (Hollett, Hassett and Lumsden, 2022)

Foster carers are child care experts who operate as co-professionals in the team which is responsible for fostered children and young people. They are trained, supervised and accountable like other professionals and, in many cases, know the children they are looking after better than any other professional. Unfortunately, as our State of the Nation's Foster Care survey of over 2,500 foster carers reinforced, foster carers are too often not treated as professionals meaning their expertise, opinions and knowledge are side-lined leading to frustration on the part of the foster carer and, very importantly, potentially poorer outcomes for the fostered young person. For the sake of the fostering system, the people who work within it and the children and young people who are being cared for by it, this must change.

(Williams, 2017)

We have these unspoken rules in social services: we must communicate in a bland, void manner when life around is anything but bland and void. We must show no emotion when life around us with these children and teenagers is 100 per cent emotion. We must show no spirit or personality. If we do, then we are breaking the rules. It must be said, an autistic foster carer is not likely going to recognise status in others. Nor are they likely to be bland and communicate the "professional" way. They will communicate the "real" way regardless of who they are dealing with. I would not be allowed to respond to the statement which was written about me with, "Okay. When you email about children's lives, or hand out your rules for them, your emails are robotic and devoid of soul, and I have issue with this". Acceptable communication is not a two-way street!

It is always easy to say we accept neurodivergent people until neurodivergent people are neurodivergent!

(An aside: This book is probably the best "nondramatic" piece of writing I have ever, or ever will have, achieved. Social services would be proud! There have been numerous edits for each chapter to tone down my "dramatic communication style"!)

Reasonable adjustments

1. Autistic foster carers need to understand the validity of rules. If rules do not make sense, then they will be questioned. You may find our questioning shows that the rule is not needed and can be deleted. It takes a strong social worker to say, "Okay, yes, this rule is gone". We need social workers who will work with us and think outside the box, seeing the bigger vision, acknowledging our 24/7 hands on experience. We will be the first to acknowledge if something we ask to try does not work and will apologise for not trusting.

2. Rules like policy and procedures for allegations need to be followed to the letter for autistic foster carers or there needs to be a believable reason, based on verifiable facts, if they are not.

3. When policy and procedures are not upheld your autistic foster carer will lose their ability to mask and present appropriately. You will see more signs of "overwhelm" and they will lose the ability to use their executive functioning skills. It will be too much for them. It becomes all too easy to twist them from being the "victim" in this situation to the "bad guy" because they are not able to cope with the bad practice, unprofessionalism, and law breaking. Let them take breaks, let them leave meetings. Hear what they actually have to say, not what you think they may be saying. Although it is not said the way you would like they most certainly will have 100 per cent valid points to make. It is only right that you as part of the social services, or as a social worker, make changes so that these negative feelings never happen again. In other words, make your policies and procedures workable, and adhere to them.

4. Think about the rules there are. If they can be broken, with or without intentional omission, I would suggest they are rules to

protect you or the organisation and not the foster carer or the child in care. The sitting on the bed rule was stated as of great importance, then we were told to ignore it. If a child had turned round and said, "I was sick last night so Anne sat on my bed and gave me a glass of water", Anne could then be in trouble even though Anne had been told it was a rule which could be broken. If Anne then said, "I was told to break the rule", I can almost certainly put two and two together and see that this information would be unreported or ignored. Social services can easily slip into self-protection mode and the "rules" help this. The question is why does the social service system, or you as a social worker, need woolly, changeable rules? Keep it simple, keep it right, or there is probably something deeper and darker going on.

5. Timeframe rules. A meeting must be X amount of time long. Why? Be flexible. Is the information you need to address really important? Do you really need to sit there for two hours? Once you have off-loaded the information there really is no need to stay. It is not rude to end a meeting with an autistic foster carer early. This will, in fact, help the autistic foster carer know that when things are done, they are done, rather than to start to feel anxious that there are another 50 minutes to sit out, without knowing why or what added value they will give.

6. Do not put our communication style down. We do not ask you to change your communication style unless we think you are using psychological abuse tactics. Work with difference not against it and it really will not be an issue. If you have an issue with our style of communication it is not the autistic foster carer's problem, it is yours. In fact, I would go so far as to say, it is a non-issue and you are using misdirection when taking issue with it.

7
Autistic overwhelm

Meltdown, shutdown, and burnout

This is the section I did not want to write. I think I have hinted at all of these in a few chapters, but they do need special attention and giving them their own chapter seems to be the correct place to talk about them. Unless the reasons for these are fully understood, autistic foster carers will continue to be shamed due to their apparently over-the-top reactions when faced with situations which cause overwhelm for them.

Meltdown

Children and adult autistics can have meltdowns. Different autistics can have meltdowns and shutdowns over different things, for example, sensory overload. However, my meltdowns happen when I am overwhelmed by injustice.

What is a meltdown?

A meltdown is an intense response to an overwhelming situation. It happens when someone becomes completely overwhelmed by their current situation and temporarily loses control of their behaviour. This loss of control can be expressed verbally (eg shouting,

> screaming, crying), physically (eg kicking, lashing out, biting) or in both ways.
> A meltdown is not the same as a temper tantrum. … When a person is completely overwhelmed, and their condition means it is difficult to express that in another way, it is understandable that the result is a meltdown. Meltdowns are not the only way an autistic person may express feeling overwhelmed. They may also refuse to interact, withdrawing from situations they find challenging or avoiding them altogether.
>
> (National Autistic Society, 2020b)

As an autistic I find it very hard to lie. If I do try it and am challenged, I will immediately admit, "Yes. I lied". And, yes, I have had my fair share of meltdowns on social services adults because there does not seem to be the same ability to admit to lying in a neurotypical.

> Lies are widely accepted, even encouraged in Western culture, neurotypical culture. People lie to avoid confrontation, to avoid taking responsibility for misbehavior, to gain power, such as jobs they don't deserve.
>
> (Collins, 2022)

My meltdowns are due to cognitive overload and happen when I am in an overwhelming position with another adult. There are many examples of these situations in this book. I have never had a meltdown with my children or teenagers, because I expect children to be children and I expect teenagers to be teenagers. Even if they try unhelpful communication tactics I am not in a position of "overwhelm". Frustrated and irritated maybe, but not overwhelmed. I expect them to try a bit of gaslighting or go for a dollop of twisting and projection. This is part of growing up and it is why we adults are there to show them what works and what does not work, and what is healthy and what is not healthy, in communication, and to teach influence over control tactics. Do not get me wrong, I am not a deity! When my child or young person lies, I will be triggered and will need to vent on my support group.

Where I cannot cope, on a meltdown level, is when adults use these tactics, the tactics found in Chapter 5. I do not expect these behaviours from them. While it is apparently alright to call these behaviours out in children, what makes it even more mind blowing is that it is not acceptable to call it out to an adult, including those in social services. As I look at the adult taking part in these behaviours I think, "You tell children off for doing this, yet you expect it to be accepted when it is you behaving like this!" The double standard is outrageous.

Because my autistic pursuit of truth and sense of justice is so heightened, I have no ability to do any of these tactics myself. In a meeting I am not able to politely say, "Can you please stop twisting what I am saying and gaslighting and stick to the truth and proven fact". The backlash if I did that would be swift and severe. So I stay quiet, it builds up inside and then I try to escape. When I am not allowed to do this either I melt down.

As adults working alongside social services, we have to pretend that the issues raised in Chapter 5 are not happening. With a child we can help them understand what they are doing. With an adult we are expected to accept it and let it happen because we are afraid of the consequences.

I was in one Teams meeting where the comments made were seriously unfair on the teenager I was fostering. The whole meeting was full of untruthful communication. The reality of the teenager's situation was not considered at any point. I said throughout the meeting words along the lines of "Please, stop. I can't do this. I can't hear you say this stuff. I can't do this. I want to leave the meeting. Write what you want but I can't sit and listen to this". I was told no, the meeting had to go ahead and I was required to stay.

I could feel the meltdown beginning to happen. It started with me crying with frustration, and apologising for crying but explaining that I could not cope with the unfair discussion regarding the teenager. I then got angry at myself for crying so I decided to watch TV during the rest of the meeting, thus distancing myself from it! As I said it was a Teams meeting which meant I could surreptitiously disengage. However, someone realised something was amiss and I was told to pay attention. I listened to more words which were used to simply cover these professionals for their unhelpful choices, making the subsequent situation the teenager's problem. It was, in fact, a social services problem. We all knew that was the case, but no one was willing to say it. I lost it. Everything in me now wants to sanitise what happened next but if we are really to understand meltdown I cannot. I cried and shouted, most likely something like, "This is bull****! You are lying, gaslighting, projecting and twisting the facts to protect yourselves and I can't believe this of you. You are better than this, I expect more from you. I am disappointed in you. I'm done, fire me. F*** this".

I left the meeting immediately. I am fully aware that those present would not have seen my outburst as "professional". Later I emailed and apologised for the meltdown. But by then I was labelled because of it. The cause was immaterial. The fact that everyone knew that, if I was in a curated truth situation, I could not cope with it, was immaterial. They knew this because I regularly told them prior to meetings, "Here's a heads up …" The fact that I had spoken the truth when no one else would was also immaterial. I had exploded and that was enough to brand me.

In a meltdown I:

- Ask to withdraw or leave.
- Say, "I can't do this".
- End up crying, swearing, and shouting the absolute irrefutable truth.
- Leave.
- Or, if still unable to leave, I refuse to interact till the meeting is over.

There is a pattern. There is a build-up. There is a warning. For me it is the internal emotional feeling of being in an unjust, unprofessional, negligent, unethical experience that triggers an outward emotional and behavioural response of the same intensity.

The meltdown is an external expression of the internal pressure build up. I know it is happening, but my resources are gone. I have tried and used all my resources to get me out of the situation to no avail. Then I melt down.

In the early years of fostering alongside social services I would find myself in shutdown after a meltdown. But then, after a fair few years, I learned to skip the meltdown phase and go straight into shutdown. It was safer for everyone else but no less harmful for me. I started fostering in my early thirties and by the time I was in my early forties I went into shutdown more often than meltdown on social services.

Shutdown

Ambitious About Autism explains the difference between meltdowns and shutdowns like this:

> Meltdowns are often the result of situations which are highly stimulating or create high levels of anxiety which feel like they can't be escaped. When someone is in this situation their reaction is either flight, fight or freeze. If the person cannot escape that leaves two options: either fight or freeze.
> Meltdowns are similar to the fight response.
> When an autistic person is having a meltdown they often have increased levels of anxiety and distress which are often interpreted as frustration, a "tantrum" or an aggressive panic attack.
> It's important to understand that meltdowns are not "temper tantrums". They are a reaction to a highly distressing situation or environment.
> If meltdowns are equivalent to the fight response, then shutdowns are similar to the freeze response.
> They are often the result of situations with high demand in one or a few of the following areas:

- social situations
- situations that require a lot of thinking
- lack of sleep
- very emotional situations
- situations that are very active or physical.

(Ambitious About Autism, n.d.)

Whenever there was a situation similar to those you will find in Chapter 5, I would feel myself getting anxious. I knew through years of experience that I would not be heard and I would not be allowed to leave and that my subsequent meltdown would be used against me. This is what a shutdown looks like in me, and in most autistics:

- disassociation,
- no resistance, no fight,
- total silence,
- full agreement regardless of what is being asked or what is heard,
- monosyllabic sentences,
- ability to form words is reduced, cannot make coherent sentences,
- more malapropisms than normal,
- heightened echolalia,
- staring into the middle distance,
- inability to look at the person or persons at all,
- physically present and mentally fully disengaged.

My whole body and mind are trying to get rid of the stress and remain calm. I just want the meeting over; I need to get out and shutdown is the best protection. I believe that from 2020 onwards

I consistently shut down. I cannot remember any meltdowns in meetings following this period in my fostering career.

When we are living daily under such conditions it is a steady route to autistic burnout. We often feel unable to continue working in a system that constantly judges us, enforces certain norms which we do not know or understand and that gives no reasonable adjustments to the way we think, reason, perceive, express, communicate, or feel.

Neurodivergent means we have a neurology that diverges from the majority.

> Neurodivergence is the term for when someone's brain processes, learns, and/or behaves differently from what is considered "typical."
> Formerly considered a problem or abnormal, scientists now understand that neurodivergence isn't inherently an issue for the individual and that it has a large societal benefit. Not all presentations of neurodivergence are a disability, like synesthesia, but all are a difference in how the brain works.
>
> (Resnick, 2023)

Our neurology is not the same as social services demands. We need to be allowed to be ourselves, then we flourish.

Trying to make us present in the way that is "expected" only results in giving autistic foster carers mental health issues.

Autistic burnout

> Autistic burnout is a syndrome conceptualised as resulting from chronic life stress and a mismatch of

expectations and abilities without adequate supports. It is characterised by pervasive, long-term (typically 3+ months) exhaustion, loss of function, and reduced tolerance to stimulus.

(Raymaker, 2022)

Autistic burnout is real and masking our autistic traits is a main reason for how it can happen. The amount of masking needed in a social situation, as we can see, is sky high. It is unachievable for many autistics. Stress, expectations we cannot reach, life changes or transitions, dismissal of our experiences, insufficient support and resources are a few of the other reasons for autistic burnout mentioned in this webpage. All are highly relevant when fostering.

Autistic burnout does not happen in a moment – it is built up over time. I knew I had to invest heavily in my self-care routines as often as possible to prevent it from happening to me.

- For as many years as I can remember I have had a massage every week. For numerous years of my time in fostering I had a massage therapist who came to my house when my children were out. She would always ask the question, "What's happened this week?" I would tell her the current issue or problem and she would help me understand what was going on, either why I was not being understood or what I was not understanding. It was like a therapy session too! She was amazing. She tried to help me understand the neurotypical world.
- I struggle with synthetic smells, but I am obsessed with aromatherapy and my home always has a calming oil diffuser on.

- I swim, do yoga, meditate and walk the dog, listen to podcasts, find ways to give my brain, which never turns off, moments to feel peace.
- I have a PhD in venting – I have a small group of close friends and, with them, there is no barrier. I overshare. I vent. I let all the emotions out, be that absolute fury to ugly crying.
- I nap. I would drop my children off at school and go back to sleep. I would plan my paid job work for the evenings so during the day I had the ability to nap and look after my child.
- Although I was a single foster carer I also had a paid job that I loved and am the founder of a charity which I love. I made sure social services was not my whole life even though social services believed they were!
- I became an advocate. I did interviews, videos, podcasts for a variety of fostering campaigns, such as The Fostering Network, "Staying Put Campaign", and went on many radio shows.

I am not perfect by any means. I also have maladaptive coping techniques. Most autistics do. But I had to plan to prevent autistic burnout. I could not burn out when I had a child in my care.

During the allegation (Chapter 6), I spent months in bed or on the sofa. For me the way this allegation was dealt with was the icing on top of the cake. I could cope with everything else, but this pushed my stress level over the edge. My burnout plan could not cover this time, or the injustice of the system which I could not fight or make right. I did not make food for myself; and, if I am honest, I did not even shower much. I did not leave my home. I did not even walk my dog; my family members did that for me. I did not speak unless I had to. I was so burnt out I could not function. I just sat or slept. Even my doctor would call to check up on me and the calls had to be taken by a family member as I could not speak to her myself. I wanted it all to end.

> According to research by Raymaker et al., there are two main factors that can contribute to autistic burnout.
>
> The *first factor (cumulative load)* is related to life stressors such as managing expectations, disabilities, work and school demands, and relationships.
>
> The *second factor (inability to obtain relief)* involves barriers to obtaining support, which may be caused by masking autistic traits, difficulties in receiving a diagnosis or accommodations, socio-economic hardships, or other people not acknowledging or understanding autistic challenges.
>
> When a person's cumulative stress is beyond the person's ability to cope, Autistic burnout sets in.
>
> (Neff, n.d.)

These two factors both peaked for me during that period. Social services knew how distressed I was by what was happening as I had told them in emails when I was trying to make them follow procedure and policy. They knew I was physically and mentally sick with autistic burnout from it. But the malpractice did not stop, as we saw. This can only be seen as abuse. To know an autistic foster carer has been so distressed by your actions and choices to the level of autistic burnout and to not fix it and make it right, even when there is no valid proof for the situation, is beyond cruel. To continue for an extra three months after it should have been over was beyond belief.

Reasonable adjustments
Meltdown

1. Your autistic foster carer probably knows what will lead to their meltdown. They will probably know what they need to ensure a meltdown does not happen. I do not have the ability to assume, so just ask them. Example: for me it is being in a curated truth situation and I need to leave.

Shutdown

2. Exactly the same as for meltdown.

Burnout

3. There should never be a time when your actions cause autistic burnout. If reasonable adjustments for the autistic foster carer are taken seriously and put in place there will probably not be autistic burnout.

Conclusion

Understanding

I spoke to a dear neurotypical friend today. They like me a lot. I like them a lot. We have walked many life miles and years together. They asked me about this book and I explained it was about "lived experience" and "reasonable adjustments". They asked for an example of a reasonable adjustment. I said, "Sometimes I would ask for something and it would be denied". They replied, "Don't you think that by asking for that you were making an issue. Couldn't you have just let it go?"

We are about to look at "understanding" but even before we can get to understanding the neurotypical has to realise their preconceived judgements and prejudices. Even a close, long-term friend of mine can think reasonable adjustments are issue-making, and if the autistic can just sit down, shut up, and deal with it, there would be no problem. And they are right. There would be no problem for the neurotypical. But the damage this mentality of "Keep the neurotypical status quo" can do to the autistic, as we have seen through this book, is immeasurable.

Awareness and understanding are not the same thing and to make a difference to autistic people's lives, it is better public understanding of autism that we need to see.

The National Autistic Society's "Too Much Information" campaign highlighted the five things autistic people have told the public they would like them to know about what it is like to be autistic:

- They need extra time to process information.
- They experience anxiety in social situations.
- They experience anxiety with unexpected changes.
- They find noise, smells, and bright lights painful and distressing.
- They become overwhelmed and experience a "meltdown" or "shutdown".

(National Autistic Society, 2018)

I hope this book has highlighted the need for understanding so that social services can shift from a verbal nod to awareness to actually understanding what autism looks like in their foster carers. Therefore, they will be able to make the reasonable adjustments that would help everyone concerned.

We hear a lot, "Don't define yourself by your autism", but this is wrong. Just as a neurotypical is defined by their neurotypicalness, we are defined by our autism. We are autistic, it is who we are. How we think, feel, and behave all stem from our brain and how our brains work. Autism is a neurodevelopmental condition. It is as impossible for us to behave, think, and feel neurotypically as it is for a fish to be a lion. It is not something we can learn or grow into.

Awareness is defined as knowledge that something exists. Awareness is not enough. We need cognitive understanding as this is the driver for change.

Stress

I found this podcast very interesting.

> Living in stress is living in survival and stress is when your brain and body are knocked out of homeostasis. Stress is when your brain and body are knocked out of balance. The stress response is what the body innately does to return itself back to balance. The problem is that if you keep turning on that fight-or-flight system, you keep turning on that emergency system, you'll actually cause people to stay out of balance and that imbalance becomes the new balance. Then they're headed for some type of disease, some type of breakdown. No organism can tolerate emergency mode for an extended period of time and when you're in survival, and that primitive system is switched on, it's really about the self. When you're in survival you have to take care of yourself.
>
> 75 to 90 percent of people that go to a health care facility in the Western World go in because of psychological or emotional stress. That's eight or nine out of ten and emotional stress and psychological stress are the ones that tend to be the most harmful because it's not T-Rex that's chasing you but it's your co-worker in the next cubicle.
>
> (Dispenza in Bartlett, 2023)

This is how it felt for me working with social services as an autistic foster carer. My children and teenagers did not cause me to live in survival mode, but the professionals did. It was constant fight or flight due to the experiences I had. Eventually over the years this imbalance became my new normal and I could not tolerate it, I had to leave. I loved fostering. I felt I was making a difference to children's lives. I had fulfilment in what I did. But I could not sustain working in the non-inclusive, neurotypical, allistic environment.

Social services need to understand the mental and emotional damage they can do to their autistic or neurodivergent foster carers.

> Research suggests that many autistic people also have a mental health problem like depression or anxiety. There are many possible reasons for this, including:
>
> - *Negative attitudes from other people.* Non-autistic people may not understand or accept your differences. You may be more likely to experience stigma, discrimination, trauma and loneliness. All these experiences contribute to mental health problems.
>
> (Mind, 2022)

The question I ask is, "Does social services want to be an organisation that does this to the people who are trying to look after their most vulnerable children?"

Empathy and double empathy issue

Dr Fung states in an article on this issue: "Most neurotypical people do not understand the world of the neurodiverse people, and vice versa" (Fung in Rosza, 2023). Because of this lack of empathy for common autistic behaviours like poor eye contact and social awkwardness, the 80 per cent of the population that is neurotypical regularly imposes on the 20 per cent that is neurodivergent "poor outcomes in both educational and employment settings".

One very common misconception about autistic people is that we lack empathy. This is completely incorrect and very dangerous. A lot of autistics have higher empathy levels than normal. For everything. I had a little mouse in my back garden which was dying. It upset me so much I got in the car and drove miles to the local animal rescue centre and made them promise me that they would save it. Now that is compassion.

I recently read that the Spanish footballer, Olga Carmona, learned after her World Cup final that her father had died on the previous Friday. This story is heartbreaking. I cried. That is empathy!

Fighting and advocating for our children and teenagers is compassion. Sympathy I have little to none of. Empathy and compassion I have in copious amounts. Compassion is empathy plus action to relieve the suffering.

If we look at empathy my question would be, "How much empathy, or compassion, (empathy in action), was I shown by the allistic social services?" From the majority of social workers, managers, and other linked professionals, absolutely zero.

> Autistic people are marginalised within society, often with limited life chances. Divides and controversies over what autism is exactly, and therefore how best to support autistic people, largely stem from the difference between seeing autism as a medicalised set of deficits to be remediated, and describing a variety of

> ways of being in the world that need accommodation and understanding. These issues have a direct bearing on what outcome measures are used in autism research and how useful they are in practice.
>
> (Milton, 2019)

From my lived experience in social services very few tried to bridge the gap with me. I have honoured those who did in this book for fairness. And when I tried to bridge the gap with social services, I was denied the opportunity.

> The autistic form of life does not conform to assumed social normativity and does not easily extend outward into the social, leading to a "double empathy problem" between people of diverse dispositions, that is, both parties struggle to understand and relate to one another. Such differences in presentation can lead to dyspathic reactions and stigma, often leading to ill-fated attempts at normalisation and a continuing vicious cycle of psycho-emotional disablement.
>
> (Milton, 2017)

There is a double empathy problem which exists between autistic people and neurotypicals.

> Simply put, the theory of the double empathy problem suggests that when people with very different experiences of the world interact with one another, they will struggle to empathise with each other.
>
> (Milton, 2018)

But again, the issue here is that autism is the protected characteristic and disability. Social services has a legal requirement to do the bridging and make reasonable adjustments. Clearly it is also important for the autistic individual to request and describe the reasonable adjustments which would help meet their needs. And when they do, they need to be listened to. The excuse of double empathy to get out of this mandated work does not hold water.

> Rather than lacking a theory of mind, it is argued here that due to differences in the way autistic people process info, they are not socialised into the same shared ethno as neurotypical people, and thus breaches in understanding happen all the time, leaving both in a state of confusion. The difference is that the neurotypical person can repair the breach, by the reassuring belief that ~99 out of 100 people still think and act like they do, and remind themselves that they are the normal ones.
>
> (Milton, 2017)

I want to shout "AMEN" when I read that quote.

Look at it this way, if I was in a wheelchair and could not walk up the steps into the office whose responsibility is it to make the reasonable adjustment? Autism, as we have seen, is a disability, so whose responsibility is it to make the reasonable adjustments for this. There is not a double empathy issue if the disability is visible. It is obvious and understood.

We would not say to the physically disabled person, "Can you stop being difficult? Get up and walk up the steps, please". We need to stop saying, in effect, to the autistic person, "Can you stop being difficult and have a neurotypical brain, please".

Equality and legality

"According to the statistics around 15 per cent to 20 per cent of the population is considered to be neurodivergent" (Embrace Consulting, 2023). Autism goes under disability; it is also a legally protected characteristic. There are going to be autistic foster carers within the system. They may be diagnosed or undiagnosed. They may have declared their disability to social services or kept the diagnosis quiet out of fear.

My local authority website says:

> The Equality Duty requires public bodies to publish information which demonstrates our due regard to:
>
> - eliminate discrimination, harassment, victimisation and any other conduct that is prohibited by or under the Equality Act 2010;
> - advance equality of opportunity between persons who share a relevant protected characteristic and persons who do not share it; and
> - foster good relations between persons who share a relevant protected characteristic and persons who do not share it.
>
> Their Equality policy: d. Ensure leadership and organisational commitment to equalities.
>
> (Local authority website. No precise source given to protect the local authority.)

I think all through this book we see discrimination, harassment, psychological abuse, and absolutely not fostering good relations between an autistic foster carer and the social services they work with.

If there is a policy, it needs to be upheld.

> The Autism Act requires workplaces to provide reasonable adjustments for autistic employees: Providing training to managers, allowing communication to take place on email, creating time for breaks and reducing sensory distractions. These are all simple steps that can be taken to make the workplace more autism friendly.
>
> (Rebello-Tindall and Tudway, 2021)

Social services social workers, managers and other linked professionals have a duty to make reasonable adjustments so neurodivergent foster carers are not at a disadvantage compared to neurotypical or allistic foster carers.

What happened to me right up until the end of 2022 when I left was not just unfair it was not legal. Social services needs to realise this. A "duty of care" is not "negotiable", it is a legal requirement.

If my fostering managers, social workers, and other linked professionals had received training, if they had made the tiny, simple, and straightforward, reasonable adjustments and inclusive supports I have put in this book, this would be a whole different story for me and for many other autistic foster carers.

Below is information taken from my diagnosis. I gave a full copy to both my fostering agency and the local authority. I wanted them to read it, to understand any issues they had with me were because of my autism and maybe talk with me and see how we could make things better. Sadly, my desire for this did not happen. Nothing changed even when they had the whole document to help them understand me. There was no difference in how things were pre- or post-diagnosis.

The passage on communication explained so much.

Communication

5.1   Ms Tanner's training as an actress means that she has good intonation, facial expressions, gesture, and eye contact. However, there is an unusual quality about the way she speaks which is more exaggerated when she is anxious or agitated.

5.2   Ms Tanner rarely asked about the examiners' thoughts or feelings. It was, however, easy to have a conversation with her and she allowed for building of ideas and exchange of views. It was sometimes difficult to maintain the turn taking and "to and fro" aspects of conversation as Ms Tanner was keen to talk and participate.

5.3   During the course of conversations with Ms Tanner there were occasional long pauses. When asked she said she was searching for the "actual truth" as she feels she is sometimes misrepresented so she checks what she is saying before she says it.

5.4   As is common with many women on the autistic spectrum, Ms Tanner is less obviously impaired in this area. Her professional training as an actress also gives her the repertoire of gestures and prosodic features of spoken language. There is however an unusual quality about her social communication which is worth noting.

Reciprocal social interaction

5.12   Ms Tanner's social communication, that is, social overtures, quality of social response and quality of rapport all had an unusual quality. Interactions were sometimes comfortable, but it was difficult to sustain due to her levels of anxiety and her unusual presentation.

5.13   In summary Ms Tanner is markedly affected in this area. She has difficulties interpreting situations and others' intent and being able to mask her feelings. Her need for authenticity and honesty, coupled with having fixed and somewhat rigid approach to life, have undoubtedly caused difficulties both socially and in the workplace.

5.14   Ms Tanner wants to develop strategies that will help her to cope with developing her confidence, overcoming her social anxiety and to deal with stress.

Two things which arose often in my fostering experience were the "[difficulties] being able to mask her feelings. Her need for authenticity and honesty". So, by 2019, social services was fully aware that if I was in a situation where curated truth was happening, I was unable to mask. Yet, when I asked to leave meetings, I was not allowed. They knew my anxiety in certain situations and still made me stay. They knew I had a need for authenticity and honesty, and still I had to sit in many inauthentic and seemingly dishonest meetings.

They also knew I had difficulty interpreting intent. I would get a feeling something was happening but would not always be able to fully express it. For example, I wrote this to try to explain my feelings regarding one particular professional:

> I do not feel that they are in line with best practice, care of the child or respect for the foster carer. I have been here many times with X and that makes me wonder, "why do I feel like I am having warning bells sound in my head and a sick feeling in my stomach every time X is involved?" If I am wrong, and there is nothing going on, then I should not be automatically checking my back and seeing ghosts where there are none. Simply on that level we have a problem that needs resolving. But if I am right, we still have a situation that needs resolving!!
>
> (Tanner, personal communication)

As you can see from this, at that time I did not have the language to state what tactic I felt was being played. I had a visceral feeling that something was not above board. In 2020, I spent a lot of time researching the tactics that are used as I needed to understand. This then gave me the language and the understanding of intent.

It is clear in this example that I would seek help for resolution. But for resolution to take place one has to acknowledge that there is something wrong, that there is intent, that there is mal or bad practice, and this is not liked. Resolution hardly ever happened and there was only denial. I would, yet again, be the one with the problem.

In the documentation of my diagnosis all my sensory issues were spelt out. I will not bore you with every page of the document but, again, this meant that everyone involved with me knew why I could not do social events, why sensory issues happened, and still none of this was talked about or considered. Certainly, no reasonable adjustments ever happened. Except for me being asked to redo my medical nothing changed in all the following years I stayed in fostering after the diagnosis.

I think one of the things for me to acknowledge is that, not only were no reasonable adjustments made, which apart from being illegal is, on a personal level, very sad. But even when I asked for a reasonable adjustment it was denied or turned against me.

We see this when I asked for one manager in particular to have email communication with me, not telephone conversations (see Chapter 5). I just wanted a reasonable adjustment, and, again, it was with one person not people in the plural. We see it when I asked to be excused from a meeting which was causing me distress and I was denied. We see it when I asked if I could stand at the back in training sessions rather than sit for four hours and it was denied. Why? Because, apparently, others would not like me "hovering at the back". We see it when I explain, "I can't do a social. I'm sorry. I am not coming". And it gets reported that I think I am special and above others to such an extent that I will not even join in!

There are so many examples I could give of asking for reasonable adjustments and being denied them right up until the end of 2022 when I realised that, for my mental health, I could no longer continue. I was so depressed by that point I was not in autistic burnout. I was now in actual mental breakdown. When I told my doctor that I was leaving fostering she replied, "I'm really pleased. This has been too damaging for you!"

As we can see from the above, many, if not all, of the difficulties and lived experiences I write about in this book did not need to have happened if the fostering social services was focused on inclusion and understanding difference. But the agenda was always to have polarised goodies and baddies.

Some statistics

> IFAs [Independent Fostering Agencies] reported a ratio of 23 initial enquiries per application [to become a foster carer] and LAs [Local Authorities] reported a ratio of 8 initial enquiries per application.
> LA services reported that 31% of mainstream fostering deregistrations were within 2 years of approval ...
> In 2021 to 2022, more mainstream fostering households deregistered (5,435) than were approved (4,035), leading to a net decrease in fostering capacity since last year.
> During 2021 to 2022, 290 households were both approved and deregistered.
> The split between the 2 sectors of all deregistrations was relatively even, with 54% (2,925) of deregistrations occurring in LAs and 46% (2,510) in IFAs.
> IFAs have seen an increase in capacity of 440 households (3%) from 2018 to 2022. The LA sector has seen a decrease in capacity of 1,770 households (8%) during the same period.
> The challenge in England is that in the last reported fiscal year (ending March 2022), more mainstream foster carers (not family and friends foster carers) stopped fostering than were approved, leading to a net decrease in fostering capacity. At the same time the number of children in care increased.
>
> (Ofsted, 2022)

These statistics show how we need foster carers – currently about 7,200 more foster carers this year alone. Yet, alarmingly, more and more foster carers are leaving each month. It is important that all aspects of this service are looked into to find out why.

What do we want in a foster carer?

I was one of the best foster carers they had. This is not a lack of humility, I am autistic. I know this because so many professionals linked to social services, that is, police or psychologists and others, told me. I have numerous children who had other foster carers after me. But once they left the social services system they continued to stay in touch. Now, even though they are in their twenties, they choose to spend Christmas Day and other events with me. This proves that I did not do too shoddy a job!

This sentence was emailed to me by a child social worker who was letting me know they were leaving social services: "I was so impressed with your connection and care of your child, your experience, and my learning will stay with me. All the best" (Child social worker, personal communication).

Here's an email from another social worker who was leaving, and I wrote to say thank you because she had been wonderful.

> Dear Megan,
> Thank you for your very kind email, which I must say brought tears to my eyes. It was great working with you and, like I always said, you are a brilliant carer! Your sacrifice, passion, commitment and resourcefulness made working with you a joyous experience. You made a difference to the lives of the young people that you

worked with by exposing them to new opportunities and fully supporting their placements with you. You persevered amidst the challenges you faced and strongly advocated on behalf of the young people, in ensuring their needs were met … I could go on!

(Social worker, personal communication)

Surely this is what matters – the foster carer's ability to connect and care for the child they have. Foster carers who are passionate, resourceful, and who support the child they look after. Foster carers who sacrifice, commit, persevere, and who advocate on the child's behalf. This is not dependent on whether they can sit in a chair correctly, attend a social event, or present neurotypically.

Furthermore, as we can see in most chapters, but especially Chapters 5 and 6, being ethical, communicating without using psychological abuse, holding truth at the core, being an advocate, fighting for what was right … all these positive attributes were turned and used against me. Are they not exactly what we want in our foster carers? These are the things fostering gains in autistic foster carers. They should be celebrated not destroyed.

My top three wishes

It is a minefield navigating a neurotypical world as an autistic woman, as neurotypicals do not think, feel, be, or behave the same as us and some of the neurotypical oddities you have are as confusing for us as we are for you! But it is your world currently simply because there are more of you. If there were more of us it would be our world and neurotypical would be the "protected characteristic" or "disability". So, because of the fall of the dice, it is you who need to make the reasonable adjustments, offer resources, for example, create forms to make accommodation requests, keep records of alleged discrimination. Also, you could explain how to find support if these reasonable adjustments are not upheld.

> Equality law recognises that achieving equality for disabled people may mean changing the way that employment is structured. This could be removing physical barriers or providing extra support for a disabled worker or job applicant. This is the duty to make reasonable adjustments. Your employer has a duty to take steps to remove, reduce or prevent the obstacles you face as a disabled worker or job applicant, where it's reasonable to do so. The employer only has to make adjustments where they are aware – or should reasonably be aware – that you have a disability.
>
> (Equality and Human Rights Commission, 2022)

These are the top three things I wished had happened.

When I first started fostering, I said it was suspected that I was autistic and that waiting for a diagnosis took years, while paying for one privately was costly. So, I would not know for a long time whether these suspicions were true, but, as a heads up, here are a few things I know are different about me. I wish then, rather than being ignored, we had worked together, had a conversation, and found some easy and simple ideas to align both sides. Many of your foster carers will not know if they are neurodivergent for the same reasons I did not back in 2011 when I started this journey.

But if they behave like it then let's assume they are it and put in reasonable adjustments.

When I did get my diagnosis, I wish there had been a meeting. I wish we had looked at the struggles I was having and worked out ways to make things better, together, rather than file the document and resume the status quo. When I asked for reasonable adjustments, I wish they had been granted. I do not think anything I asked for was unfair, excessive, or required too much effort. Yet if they had been granted my mental health would not have been damaged to the point where I needed to leave this toxic environment. The environment would not have been a problem, and I could have stayed fostering, doing something I loved so much.

These simple wishes could have made this a win-win situation for both sides. And when the social workers, managers, and other linked professionals work with autistic foster carers who else wins? The child or teenager in the foster carer's care. Surely, the child or teenager is the most important person in this equation.

"Autists are the ultimate square pegs, and the problem with pounding a square peg into a round hole is not that the hammering is hard work. It's that you're destroying the peg" (Collins, 2004).

We can make fostering a beautiful and superb place for autistic foster carers to thrive. Do not destroy us. We have so much to offer, not just our loyalty, commitment, and ability to care for our nation's most vulnerable children and teenagers, but also so many other assets, including outside of the box thinking, hyper-focus, tenacity, creativity, advocacy, trust, truth, and, importantly in social services, fun!

The reasonable adjustments in this book are not difficult, costly, or time-consuming. Sit down with your autistic foster carer and just ask them what they need. They will let you know, and then add that in. Something as simple as this can change everything for the better for everyone. But, as Yoda says, "Do or do not. There is no try".

I gave everything, even my mental health. I stayed and kept trying till it became too damaging for me and I had autistic burnout and mental breakdown.

One of my favourite songs, "You're the Voice", by John Farnham (1986), is such a song for unity, even though it was written as a protest song. On both of these counts it is similar to this book:

> We have the chance to turn the pages over.
> We can write what we want to write.
> We gotta make ends meet, before we get
>   much older
> This time, we know we all can stand together.
> With the power to be powerful
> Believing we can make it better.
> Ooh, we're all someone's daughter.
> We're all someone's son.
> How long can we look at each other,
> Down the barrel of a gun?
> You're the voice, try and understand it.
> Make a noise and make it clear,
> We're not gonna sit in silence.
> We're not gonna live with fear.

Can autistic foster carers and social services unite? Can you allow difference? Can you see the value we autistic foster carers add? Can we stand together, make it better, write a new way?

I hope this book never needs to be written again. It should not have needed to be written in the first place. And, no, child social worker 2022, there is nothing wrong with me! Remember: "When you see something that is not right, not just, not fair, you have a moral obligation to say something, to do something" (Lewis, remarks on the House floor during the impeachment of President Donald Trump, December 2019).

Recommended assignments and discussion questions

What makes "difference" frightening? Why may we have difficulties with neurodivergent behaviours or communication?

Watch this Ted Talk: www.youtube.com/watch?v=Qvvrme5WiwA. Hold in mind this book while watching. Make decisions on all the ways you can hold space for difference and create inclusion for your neurodivergent foster carers.

For each chapter in this book consider how neurotypical your thinking is. What are your expectations on conformity and do your "necessary" beliefs add to unnecessary division and exclusion? Discuss. Being self-aware is the only way we can overcome these issues.

References

Alloway, T. (2020). Autism and Memory: Can you Guess the Memory Superpowers of a Child with Autism? Available at: www.psychologytoday.com/gb/blog/keep-it-in-mind/202004/autism-and-memory [Accessed June 2023].

Ambitious About Autism (n.d.). *Meltdowns and Shutdowns* [online]. Available at: www.ambitiousaboutautism.org.uk/information-about-autism/behaviour/meltdowns-and-shutdowns [Accessed June 2023].

Arky, B. (2023). Why Many Autistic Girls Are Overlooked. *Child Mind Institute* [online]. Available at: https://childmind.org/article/autistic-girls-overlooked-undiagnosed-autism/ [Accessed July 2023].

The Autistic Life (2021). Can You Relate? [Instagram] 19 April 2021. Available at: www.instagram.com/p/CN3FuLTM6fu [Accessed June 2023].

Australian Human Rights Commission (2023). Reasonable Adjustments [online]. Available at: https://humanrights.gov.au/quick-guide/12084 [Accessed August 2023].

Auticon (2023). Autism Influences a Person's Perception, Cognition, and Emotions [online]. Available at: https://auticon.com/autism/ [Accessed June 2023].

Bartlett, S. (2023). "Doctor Joe Dispenza: Your Thoughts Are Making You Sick! You MUST Do This Before 10am to Fix It!", *The Diary of a CEO with Steven Bartlett* [Podcast]. 14 August 2023. Available at: https://podcasts.apple.com/gb/podcast/doctor-joe-dispenza-your-thoughts-are-making-you-sick/id1291423644?i=1000624351371 [Accessed August 2023].

Bennie, M. (2018). Executive Function: What Is It, and How Do We Support It in Those with Autism? Pt 1 [online]. Available at: https://autismawarenesscentre.com/executive-function-what-is-it-and-how-do-we-support-it-in-those-with-autism-part-i/ [Accessed June 2023].

Brinkert, J. and Remington, A. (2020). Making Sense of the Perceptual Capacities in Autistic and Non-Autistic Adults. *NIH: National Library of Medicine* [online]. Available at: https://pubmed.ncbi.nlm.nih.gov/32476432/ [Accessed June 2023].

CAR Autism Roadmap (2020). Time Management and Other Executive Functioning Issues in the Workplace [online]. Available at: https://research.chop.edu/car-autism-roadmap/time-management-and-other-executive-functioning-issues-in-the-workplace [Accessed August 2023].

Ciampi, M. (2019). The Dark Side of Autism in the Workplace [online]. Available at: www.linkedin.com/pulse/dark-side-autism-workplace-marcelle-ciampi/ [Accessed June 2023].

Collins, N. (2022). Honesty Is Authenticity [online]. Available at: www.theautismcoach.co.uk/blog/honesty-is-authenticity [Accessed June 2023].

Collins, P. (2004). *Not Even Wrong: Adventures in Autism*. New York: Bloomsbury.

Cope, R. and Remington, A. (2022). The Strengths and Abilities of Autistic People in the Workplace. *Autism Adulthood*, 4(1), pp. 22–31. Available at: https://pubmed.ncbi.nlm.nih.gov/36605563/ [Accessed August 2023].

Courchesne, E. and Pierce, K. (2005). Brain Overgrowth in Autism during a Critical Time in Development: Implications for Frontal Pyramidal Neuron and Interneuron Development and Connectivity. *International Journal of Developmental Neuroscience*, 23, pp. 153–170.

Diamond, A. (2013). Executive Functions. *Annual Review of Psychology,* [online] 64, pp. 135–168. Available at: www.ncbi.nlm.nih.gov/pmc/articles/PMC4084861/ [Accessed August 2023].

Dictionary.com (n.d.). Misdirection [online]. Available at: www.dictionary.com/browse/misdirection [Accessed June 2023].

"Doublespeak", (2023). Wikipedia [online]. Available at: https://en.wikipedia.org/wiki/Doublespeak [Accessed August 2023].

Embrace Consulting (2023). What Percentage Do You Think Is Neurodivergent? [online]. Available at: www.linkedin.com/pulse/what-percentage-do-you-think-neurodivergent-embraceconsulting/ [Accessed August 2023].

Equality and Human Rights Commission (2022). In Employment: Workplace Adjustments [online]. Available at: www.equalityhumanrights.com/en/multipage-guide/employment-workplace-adjustments [Accessed June 2023].

Farnham, J. (1986), 'You're the Voice', *Whispering Jack* [CD]. Melbourne, Australia: Wheatley.

Foster Care Workers Union (n.d.). *Making Change.* Available at: www.fosteriwgb.co.uk/change [Accessed June 2023].

Foster Support (2022). *National Fostering Association Consortium* [online]. Available at: www.fostersupport.co.uk/national-fostering-association-consortium [Accessed July 2023].

The Fostering Network (2021). *State of the Nation's Foster Care 2021 Thematic Report 2: Allegations* [online]. Available at: https://thefosteringnetwork.org.uk/sites/default/files/2022-04/State%20of%20the%20Nation%20Thematic%20report%202%20Allegations_0.pdf [Accessed June 2023].

FosterWiki (2021). *Top 10 Tips: Your Information and Data* [online]. Available at: https://fosterwiki.com/wiki/top-10-tips-your-information-and-data/ [Accessed June 2023].

Gadsby, H. (2020). How Hannah Gadsby's High-Functioning Autism Works. Netflix Is a Joke. YouTube. Available at: www.youtube.com/watch?v=5IXbpgU9OWk [Accessed August 2023].

Gajanan, M. (2017). 11 of Michelle Obama's Most Inspiring, Empowering Quotes [online]. Available at: https://time.com/4639410/michelle-obama-best-quotes/ [Accessed July 2023].

Gatfield, O., Hall, G., Isaacs, K. and Mahony, J. (2018). Guidelines for Creating Autistic Inclusive Environments [online]. Available at: www.autismcrc.com.au/sites/default/files/inline-files/Guidelines%20for%20Creating%20Autistic%20Inclusive%20Environments%20(002).pdf [Accessed August 2023].

Hollett, M., Hassett, A. and Lumsden, V. (2022). Foster Caring as 'Professional Parenting': A Grounded Theory of The Relationships Between Parent and Professional in Long-term Foster Care. *Sage Journals – Adoption and Fostering* [online]. Available at: https://journals.sagepub.com/doi/10.1177/03085759221139490 [Accessed June 2023].

Hopper, G. M. (1987). Interview in *InformationWeek*, 9 March 1987, p. 52.

Huston, M. (2021). Are Autistic People Empathic? Is Everyone Else? *Psychology Today Australia* [online]. Available at: www.psychologytoday.com/au/blog/everyday-neurodiversity/202101/are-autistic-people-empathic-is-everyone-else [Accessed June 2023].

Jack, C. (2022). 'Why Autistic People Can Struggle in the Workplace'. *Psychology Today* [online]. Available at: www.psychologytoday.com/gb/blog/women-autism-spectrum-disorder/202211/why-autistic-people-can-struggle-in-the-workplace [Accessed June 2023].

Koshino, H., et al. (2005). Functional Connectivity in an fMRI Working Memory Task in High-Functioning Autism. *Neuroimage*, 24, pp. 810–821.

Li, H., et al. (2022). *Comprehensive Clinical Psychology*. 2nd ed. [online] Available at: www.sciencedirect.com/topics/psychology/inhibitory-control [Accessed June 2023].

Luna, B., Minshew, N. J., Garver, K. E., Lazar, N. A., Thulborn, K. R., Eddy, W. F. and Sweeney, J. (2002). Neocortical System Abnormalities in Autism: An fMRI Study of Spatial Working Memory. *Neurology*, 59, pp. 834–840.

McNulty, J. (2018). Autistic People Want to Socialize: They Just May Show It Differently. University of California [online]. Available at: www.universityofcalifornia.edu/news/autistic-people-want-socialize-they-just-may-show-it-differently [Accessed June 2023].

Merriam-Webster Dictionary (2023). Executive Function. Available at: www.merriamwebster.com/dictionary/executive%20function [Accessed June 2023].

Milton, D. (2017). *A Mismatch of Salience*. Teddington, UK: Pavilion Publishing.

Milton, D. (2018). The Double Empathy Problem [online]. *National Autistic Society*. Available at: www.autism.org.uk/advice-and-guidance/professional-practice/double-empathy [Accessed June 2023].

Milton, D. (2019). Beyond Tokenism: Autistic People in Autism Research [online]. *British Psychological Society*. Available at: www.bps.org.uk/psychologist/beyond-tokenism-autistic-people-autism-research [Accessed June 2023].

Mind (2022). Autism and Mental Health [online]. Available at: www.mind.org.uk/about-us/our-policy-work/equality-and-human-rights/autism-and-mental-health/ [Accessed August 2023].

Miserandino, C. (2003). The Spoon Theory [online]. Available at: https://butyoudontlooksick.com/ [Accessed June 2023].

National Autistic Society (2018). Too Much Information [online]. Available at: www.autism.org.uk/what-we-do/campaign/public-understanding/too-much-information [Accessed June 2023].

National Autistic Society (2020a). *Dealing with Change: A Guide for All Audiences* [online]. Available at: www.autism.org.uk/advice-and-guidance/topics/behaviour/dealing-with-change/all-audiences [Accessed June 2023].

National Autistic Society (2020b). *Meltdowns: A Guide for All Audiences* [online]. Available at: www.autism.org.uk/advice-and-guidance/topics/behaviour/meltdowns/all-audiences [Accessed July 2023].

National Autistic Society (2023). Support at Work: A Guide for Autistic People Institute [online]. Available at: www.autism.org.uk/advice-and-guidance/topics/employment/support-at-work/autistic-adults [Accessed July 2023].

National Bullying Helpline (2022). Gaslighting at Work. Spotting the Signs of Subtle Workplace Bullying [online]. Available at: www.nationalbullyinghelpline.co.uk/gaslighting.html [Accessed June 2023].

Neff, M. (n.d.). What Causes Autistic Burnout? How to Identify Root Causes. *Neurodivergent Insights* [online]. Available at: https://neurodivergentinsights.com/blog/what-causes-autistic-burnout [Accessed June 2023].

Ofsted (2022). Fostering in England 1 April 2021 to 31 March 2022 [online]. Available at: www.gov.uk/government/statistics/fostering-in-england-1-april-2021-to-31-march-2022/fostering-in-england-1-april-2021-to-31-march-2022 [Accessed June 2023].

Praslova, L. (2022). Workplace Bullying of Autistic People: A Vicious Cycle [online]. Available at: https://us.specialisterne.com/workplace-bullying-of-autistic-people-a-vicious-cycle/ [Accessed July 2023].

Raymaker, D. (2022). Understanding Autistic Burnout. *National Autistic Society* [online]. Available at: www.autism.org.uk/advice-and-guidance/professional-practice/autistic-burnout [Accessed July 2023].

Rebello-Tindall, M. and Tudway, J. (2021). 12 Things Autistic People Want You to Know This World Autism Awareness Week. *Dimensions* [online]. Available at: https://dimensions-uk.org/press-release/12-things-autistic-people-want-you-to-know/ [Accessed June 2023].

Resnick, A. (2023). What Does It Mean to Be Neurodivergent? [online]. Available at: www.verywellmind.com/what-is-neurodivergence-and-what-does-it-mean-to-be-neurodivergent-5196627 [Accessed July 2023].

Rosza, M. (2023). 'Neurotypicals: What Makes Them Tick, and How Can Autistic People Better Understand Them?' *Salon* [online]. Available at: www.salon.com/2023/06/05/neurotypical-people-explainer [Accessed August 2023].

Rudy, L. (2022). Echolalia [online]. Available at: www.verywellhealth.com/echolalia-5224088 [Accessed June 2023].

Tanner, M. (2020). *NVR: Nonviolent Resistance* [online]. Think NVR. Available at: www.thinknvr.co.uk/about-nvr [Accessed June 2023].

Williams, K. (2017). It's Time to Treat Foster Carers as the Professionals that they are. *The Fostering Network* [online]. Available at: www.thefosteringnetwork.org.uk/blogs/kevin-williams/its-time-treat-foster-carers-professionals-they-are [Accessed July 2023].

Recommended further reading

YouTube TED talks on autism – various speakers.

Auticon. Autism: *In Conversation with Auticon* [Podcast]. Available at: https://podcasts.apple.com/gb/podcast/autism-in-conversation-with-auticon/id1595836489

Spotify. https://open.spotify.com/show/2rVNtrqcptuar4leOaxZa0

Price, D. (2022). *Unmasking Autism*. London: Monoray.

Glossary

Assessing Social Worker

The social worker who does the Form F.

CAMHS

Child and Adolescent Mental Health Services: This is an NHS (National Health Service) service that assesses and treats children and adolescents if there are emotional, behavioural, or mental health difficulties. CAMHS professionals include therapists, psychologists, nurses, psychiatrists, social workers, and support workers.

Child Social Worker

The social worker who looks after the child.

Form F

Prospective Foster Carer Report (Form F) England. "In essence, an assessment using Form F is primarily about identifying whether an applicant or applicants are suitable to be approved as foster carers, to determine the kind of fostering for which they are suitable, and to consider any terms of approval. The form offers a structure for providing evidence about these matters to fostering panels and to fostering service decision-makers." https://corambaaf.org.uk/sites/default/files/electronic-forms/SAMPLE%20CoramBAAF%20Form%20F%20(England)%202019.pdf

This takes around 3 to 6 months to complete. It is a long document full of questions about everything to do with the foster carer's history. An assessing social worker comes to your home for many visits and you talk through your whole life.

Foster Carer Medical

This is a form that needs to be filled out prior to acceptance as a foster carer. We revisit the medical every three years. Our GP (general practitioner) also has a form to fill out. The questions are on health and lifestyle and current physical and mental health. The GP does not offer an opinion on the suitability to foster, they just give factual answers to the questions posed. The form then gets sent back to the local authority and or the independent fostering agency.

Independent Fostering Agency or Agency (IFA)

Independent fostering agency: agencies work alongside the local authority and provide foster carers and foster carer support. I worked for my local authority for some years as a foster carer and then transferred to an IFA. Foster carers can switch from one to another.

IRO

Independent Reviewing Officers (IROs) are social workers, who are also required to be experienced social work managers. Local authorities have a duty to appoint an IRO to every child in care. IROs are required to oversee and scrutinise the care plan of the child/young person and ensure that everyone who is involved in the life of that child/young person fulfils his or her responsibilities. https://nairo.org.uk/about/what-is-an-iro/

Journey to Foster

Journey to Foster is a pre-approval training course written by experienced social workers for pre-approval of foster carers. Prospective carers will learn the fundamentals of becoming a foster carer and what the role entails, the concept of attachment, welcoming a child into the home for the first time, and promoting positive relationships with the team around the child and birth family members. Every foster carer has to do this course. It is generally two or three days long. It can be virtual or face to face. https://fostertalk.org/training-course-journey-2-fosters

LAC Meeting

Looked After Child Review: Generally LAC meetings take place every six months. All the professionals who are involved with the child come together to review the child's care plan, talk about how things are going, and decide what might need to be done next.

Linked Professionals

In the book I call any professional who is not a social worker a "linked professional". They may be a doctor, psychologist, CAMHS professional, member of the police, etc.

Local Authority (LA)

This is the council in the district where you live that is responsible for any children taken into care. The local authority will place children with their own foster carers or with foster carers from an agency. The child social worker is always from the local authority. The supervising social worker will be from the local authority if you foster through them or with the independent fostering agency if you foster with an agency.

Logs

These are daily, weekly, or monthly reports on the child in their care which are sent to social workers and must be completed by the foster carer. Information is added under headings such as education, social wellbeing, emotional wellbeing, life skills, safeguarding issues.

PEP Meeting

Personal Education Plan: This meeting is concerned with the child's education, how things are going in school and what extra support might be needed. The child social worker, teachers, foster carers all attend, and CAMHS personnel may be there if required.

Supervising Social Worker

The social worker who looks after the foster carer.

Index

accountability 90
agency fostering authority 61
allegations 61, 64, 87, 108
   policy surrounding 88
anxiety 18
attitude problem 4, 15
autism
   benefits 1
   characteristics xvii, 3, 6–7, 21, 26, 43–45, 47, 52
   in childhood x
   cognitive strengths 9
   definition 112
   diagnosis ix
   misconceptions 115
   negative attitudes towards 114
   understanding of xi
Autism Act 119
autistic foster carer
   benefits of 1
   in social services 79
autistic overwhelm
   burnout 106
   meltdown 99
   shutdown 104

body language 20–21
brain development 12
burnout *see* autistic overwhelm, burnout

child sexual exploitation xvi
children
   rules on 92
   safeguarding 86
communication 120,
   behaviour as 4
   email 66
   face and body for 20
   problem and misrepresentation 63
   rule 94
   tactics 100
   techniques xiii
   written 65
cumulative load 109

defiance xvi
detail errors 11

difference x, 7
different initial premises 18
discrimination 7
double empathy 117
dysregulation xvi

echolalia 28
emotion 60, 62
   abuse 82
   damage 114
   reality 4
empathy 51
   and double empathy issue 114
Equalities Act 2010 xvii
equality, and legality 118
executive functioning differences 44
   definition of 31
   impulse inhibition 36
   planning and organisation 34
   reasonable adjustments 38
   staying focused 35
   time management 37
   working memory 33
executive functions (EFs)
   definition of 31
expectations 107

facial expression 21

facial language 20
foster carer
   appreciation 53
   community x
   retention of xvii
foster child
   relationship with 71
fostering agency 35

Gadsby, Hannah 28
gaslighting 61
grief 62

happiness 53
historical allegation 88, 91
humour
   contrived forms of 27
   sense of 8–9, 26
   social interaction 27

impulse inhibition behaviours 37
information
   words for 50
inhibitory control 36
intentional omissions 67
IRO (independent reviewing officer) 66

judgements 6

labelling 72
legality, equality and 118
lies 100

masking 17
meltdown *see* autistic overwhelm, burnout
memory 25
mental damage 114
Miserandino, Christine 44

name calling 69
National Autistic Society xvii
neurodivergence ix, 12, 106
neurotypicals 20, 22
Nineteen Eighty-Four (Orwell) 59
non-autistic person 33
non-violent resistance (NVR) parenting 2, 12

Obama, Michelle xviii
omissions, intentional 67
organisation 39
Orwell, George 59
overwhelm *see* autistic overwhelm

parenting xvi
parents 4–7
perceptual capacity 46

planning 39
predetermined expectations 22
professionals 10
projection 15
psychological abuse 82

reasonable adjustments 16, 30, 65, 111
reciprocal social interaction 121
relationship 6
rule differences
  description of 85
  general rules on children or teenagers 92
  policy and procedure rules 87
  timeframe rules 93

self-harm xvi
sensory aspect 46
sensory overload 37
shoe gate 6
shutdown *see* autistic overwhelm, shutdown
single carer fostering 45
small talk 48
smells 47
social care xi, xvi
social care professionals 66
social communication 16

social demands 44
social differences
 gossip 50
 info-dumping 50
 sensory aspect 46
 small talk 48
 social aspect of fostering 43
 social hangover 45
 spoon theory 44
 words for information 50
social hangover 45
social interaction 16
social occasion 46
social service manager 7, 67
social services xi, xviii, 54, 67, 79, 82, 112, 116
 "status-driven" organisation 95
social worker v, 68
 celebration of xii
 expectation 22
social workers xv
sound 47
spoon theory 44
State of the Nation's Foster Care survey 95
stimuli, behavioural responses to 36
stress 105, 107, 113
 levels of living xiv

supervising social worker xiii, 4, 17, 34–35, 52
survival mode xv
sustained perseverance 11

teenagers 8, 13, 92, 102
timeframe rules 93
time management 37
touch 47
triangulation 67
truth differences
 changing minds 72
 description of 59
 gaslighting 61
 intentional omissions 67
 labelling 72
 misdirection 77
 name calling 69
 projection 15
 theories treated as fact 70
 triangulation 67
 twisting 65
 using threats or coercion 75

verifiable facts 75
vestibular hypersensitivity 48
visual 47

working memory 33, 38

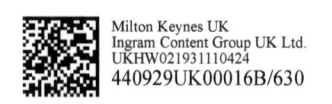

Milton Keynes UK
Ingram Content Group UK Ltd.
UKHW021931110424
440929UK00016B/630

9 781915 734716